Immunological Screening and Immunotherapy in Critically ill Patients with Abdominal Infections

W0114876

Springer

Berlin
Heidelberg
New York
Barcelona
Hong Kong
London
Milan
Paris
Singapore
Tokyo

E. Faist (Ed.)

Immunological Screening and Immunotherapy in Critically ill Patients with Abdominal Infections

With 41 Figures and 35 Tables

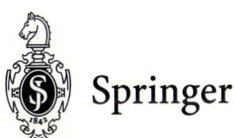 Springer

FAIST, E., Professor Dr. med.
Chirurgische Universtität der LMU München
Klinikum Großhadern
Marchioninistraße 15
81377 München

ISBN 3-540-41148-8 Springer-Verlag Berlin Heidelberg New York

CIP data applied for

Immunological screening and immunotherapy in critically ill patients with abdominal infections ; with 35 tables / Eugen Faist. - Berlin ; Heidelberg ; New York ; Barcelona ; Hong Kong ; London ; Mailand ; Paris ; Singapore ; Tokyo : Springer, 2001
ISBN 3-540-41148-8

Springer-Verlag Berlin Heidelberg New York
a member of BertelsmannSpringer Science+Business Media GmbH

http://www.springer.de

© Springer-Verlag Berlin Heidelberg 2001
Printed in Germany

Typesetting: Fotosatz-Service Köhler GmbH, Würzburg
Cover design: design & production GmbH, Heidelberg
Printed on acid-free paper   SPIN 10780165   18/3130/ag   5 4 3 2 1 0

Preface

Over two decades an abundance of knowledge has been accumulated focusing on the understanding of the molecular and cellular pathomechanisms of stressful conditions like systemic inflammation and sepsis.

We have learned that there is a clear correlation between the magnitude of the inciting traumatic event and the degree of inflammatory dysbalance.

The immunoinflammatory disintegration comprises a simultaneous collapse of the otherwise very smoothly balanced pro- and antiinflammatory vectors of cytokine regulation.

Most recently, we understood that it is predominantly the dysregulation of antiinflammatory mediators that plays a pivotal role for the phenomenon of trauma-induced depression or paralysis of cell-mediated immune responses.

The substantial intellectual and logistic investments of numerous investigators towards understanding the biology of sepsis inevitably lead us towards a rewarding status in terms of reaching spheres of clinical relevance. From the evolutionary collection of a multitude of ex-vivo and in-vivo immuno-mechanistic parameters, some were found to represent most significant biological markers to support the clinician to characterize better the severity of inflammatory illness and to predict outcome.

Chapter one of this book, authored by G. Grass and E.A.M. Neugebauer, analyses elegantly our current knowledge on the assessment of the immunological status in terms of risk and prognosis of sepsis.

Further on, many of us who have done research in the field of assessing biochemical parameters agree that the availability of a strong, reliable and pragmatic immunomonitoring system represents the crucial precondition to develop reasonable and responsible modes of preventive and interventive immunomodulatory therapeutic strategies. For the successful protection of the host against progressive inflammatory dysregulation resulting in fatal multiple organ dysfunction, adjunctive immunotherapy might strengthen our armament of therapeutic interventions in the critically ill.

In chapter two, H.B. Reith and U. Mittelkötter describe their experience with the value of biological markers of inflammation to characterize the severity of abdominal sepsis which might result in a consecutive indication for the therapeutic intervention with intravenous immunoglobulins.

As it is a major focus of this book to describe the association between immunologic screening and immunotherapy in critically ill patients predominantly following intraabdominal surgery and peritonitis, chapter three, authored by M. Trautmann and P. M. Lepper, offers important information on the underlying facets of microbiology as a crucial cornerstone of diagnosis and therapy of intraabdominal infections.

In chapter four E. Hanisch and A. Encke extensively describe their work to better characterize different degrees of inflammatory morbidity in patients undergoing abdominal surgery using the definitions of SIRS and sepsis as they have been suggested by the consensus conference of the American College of Chest Physicians and the Society of Critical Care Medicine.

Finally, in chapter five, H.G. Kress reflects about limitations, pitfalls and flaws of therapeutic trials with immunotherapy. He is discussing the problems with the heterogeneity of study populations, the difficult complex of primary and surrogate endpoints as well as other crucial factors important for the value of therapeutic studies, determinants that might be responsible for the fact that our search for a magic bullet for treating inflammation and sepsis has so far been unsuccessful. It is impossible to predict where the next breakthrough will occur in the attempt to control an overwhelming inflammatory reactivity and altered host immune responses.

I express my thanks to my colleagues for their contributions to this book. I do hope that more frequent prevention of organ failure in patients with abdominal infections will result from this information.

I am most indebted to the editorial staff of Springer-Verlag, especially Mr. Thomas Günther, for their willingness and enthusiastic support in preparing this work. Finally, I would also like to thank Biotest Pharma, here Dr. Reinhard Schweitzer, for the great effort to initiate and sponsor the creation and production of this comprehensive text book.

Munich, January 2001   Prof. Dr. EUGEN FAIST, FACS
                                              Ludwig-Maximilians-University Munich
                                              Klinikum Großhadern
                                              Department of Surgery

Table of Contents

List of Contributors

ENCKE, A., Professor Dr. med.
Klinikum der Johann-Wolfgang-Goethe Univiversität
Klinik für Allg.- u. Gefäßchirurgie
Theodor-Stern-Kai 7
60590 Frankfurt

FAIST, E., Professor Dr. med.
Chirurgische Universität der LMU München
Klinikum Großhadern
Marchioninistraße 15
81377 München

GRASS, G., Dr. med.
Biochemical and Experimental Division II
Chirurgische Abteilung
Universität Köln
Ostmerheimer Straße 200
51109 Köln

HANISCH, M., Professor Dr. Dr. med.
Chirurgische Klinik
am Knappschaftskrankenhaus Dortmund
Wieckesweg 27
49309 Dortmund

KRESS, H.-G., Professor Dr. med.
Abt. für Anästhesie und Intensivmedizin B
Allg. Krankenhaus Wien
Währinger-Gürtel 18–20
A-1090 Wien
Österreich

LEPPER, P. M.
Abt. für Mikrobiologie und Hygiene
Universität Ulm
Steinhövel Str. 9
89075 Ulm

NEUGEBAUER, E. A. M., Professor Dr. med.
Biochemical and Experimental Division II
Chirurgische Abteilung
Universität Köln
Ostmerheimer Straße 200
51109 Köln

REITH, H. B., Professor Dr. med.
Chirurgische Abteilung
Universitätsklinik Würzburg
Josef-Schneider-Str. 2
97080 Würzburg

TRAUTMANN, M., Professor Dr. med.
Abt. für Mikrobiologie und Hygiene
Universität Ulm
Steinhövel Str. 9
89075 Ulm

Risk and Prognosis of Sepsis
Current Methods on the Assessment
of the Immunological Status

G. GRASS and E. A. M. NEUGEBAUER

1.1
Introduction

Despite decades of research new therapeutic strategies have failed so far to improve mortality of patients with systemic inflammatory response syndrome (SIRS) and sepsis in controlled clinical trials. The reasons for this have been discussed in symposia, workshops and a myriad of publications. There is agreement that beside relying on insufficient experimental data and wrong concepts methodological shortcomings are common (Neugebauer et al. 1998). Due to the unsuccessful trials interest shifted from therapy to prophylaxis and/or very early therapy of sepsis: "We should spend more time searching how to achieve an accurate prognosis and less time searching for a magic bullet." (Barclay 1995) Measuring the immunestatus of patients should help to identify patients at risk for up-coming prophylactic approaches or septic patients who may benefit from immunomodulatory therapies.

The human immune system is a highly complex system of interacting cells, tissues and mediators involving the whole body. Immune reactions occur locally as well as systemically. Therefore the term "imunological status" of patients can not be defined without relation to the disease and to the aim of categorizing different disease states.

The expression "systemic inflammatory response syndrome" reflects the idea that the disease formerly called sepsis or sepsis syndrome is independent of the underlying cause. It has been assumed that SIRS is the result of the dysbalance of pro- and anti-inflammatory forces (Bone 1996a). Compensatory anti-inflammatory response (CARS) is assumed to lead to an increased susceptibility to infection or anergy. Systemic spillover of the pro-inflammatory system leads to apoptosis, organ dysfunction, thus septic shock. According to this paradigm SIRS and sepsis are diseases of the immune system rather than simple effects of a causative agent. Identification of these different immunestates may be crucial for treatment of patients. When SIRS predominates anti-inflammatory therapies may be useful, whereas agents such as granulocyte colony-stimulating factor, interferon-gamma, and interleukin-13 can be used for stimulation of the immunesystem in patients with CARS.

1.2
Evaluation of Risk Factors Predisposing to Bacterial Infections and Sepsis

Preoperative Risk Factors

Risk is the probability that something negative will happen. Risk factors are parameters associated with the risk to develop a disease or complications. Preoperative risk factors may be identifiable before patients undergo surgery. Careful evaluation of these factors should influence the indication for surgery and – where applicable – the surgical technique applied.

Assessing the general health condition of patients is routinely performed. It includes age and sex, patient history and basic diagnostic procedures. It has been demonstrated that critical assessment for selecting patients to undergo major surgery improves morbidity (such as infectious complications) and mortality (Bartels et al. 1998).

The importance of the risk factor sex has first been discovered in animal experiments. Sexual hormones are potent regulators of various immune functions. Although androgens are immunosuppressive, estrogens protect against septic challenges in animal models. Best et al. found as early as 1984 that male rabbits show an enhanced susceptibility to infection (Best et al. 1984). Zellweger et al. (Zellweger et al. 1997) discovered that female rats in proestrus state maintain splenic immune functions and tolerate sepsis better than males. In recent years it became evident that the incidence of septic complications is lower in females (especially before menopause) (Wichmann et al. 1998). Male patients tend to increased production of pro-inflammatory cytokines (IL-6, TNF-α) (Majetschak et al. 2000). Moreover women do have a better prognosis in septic diseases. Oberholzer et al. (Oberholzer et al. 2000) found that the incidence of posttraumatic sepsis in severely injured patients and multiple organ dysfunction syndrome is increased in males although females did not differ with regard to injury severity. In a prospective study of sepsis mortality of female surgical

Table 1. Clinical parameters identified as risk factors

Risk factor	Evidence	Reference
Age	+	(Kawakami et al. 1999, Tang et al. 1993)
Sex	+	(Best et al. 1984, Zellweger et al. 1997, Wichmann et al. 1998, Oberholzer et al. 2000, Schröder et al. 1998)
Malnutrition	+	(Pittet et al. 1993, Chandra 1996)
Diabetes mellitus	+	(Leibovici et al. 1991, Rubio Felix et al. 1998)
Trauma	+	(Faist et al. 1986, Staphan 1987)
Antibiotics	(+)	(Taber et al. 1987, Orman et al. 2000)
Catecholamines	(+)	(van der Poll et al. 1996, Bergmann et al. 1999, Burns et al. 1997)
Corticosteroids	–/(+)[1]	(Meduri et al. 1998, Sprung 1998, Spijkstra and Girbes 2000, Sauerland et al. 2000)

Clinical parameters identified as risk factors: + clinical and experimental data, (+) experimental data but clinical data controversial or missing, – no sufficient evidence; [1] possibly beneficial effects.

patients was 26% in contrast to 70% in male patients although patients did not significantly differ according to APACHE II scoring or age (Schröder et al. 1998).

An important observation in elderly patients is their susceptibility to infection (Kawakami et al. 1999). Immunefunction declines with age, leading to increased infection and cancer rates in aged individuals. This is mainly characterized by a progressive appearance of immune dysregulation although innate immunity is preserved during the aging process (Lesuord and Mazari 1999). Environmental factors, such as nutrition, medication intake or physical activity leading to secondary immune dysfunction have to be taken into account. Especially in patients with fungemia age has been identified as an independent risk factor (Tang et al. 1993). The risk factor age is reflected by its impact in common scoring systems such as Acute Physiology Age Chronic Health Evaluation (APACHE II and III), Simplified Acute Physiology Score (SAPS) and SAPS II or Mortality Probability Models (MPM II).

Without doubt preexisting diseases do have an impact on the incidence of bacterial infections, sepsis and outcome of septic patients. Malnutrition and alcohol abuse are both independent risk factors for bacterial infections (Pittet et al. 1993, Chandra 1996). The relationship between nutrition and resistance to infection is obvious by clinical observations since the historical times of pestilence. Most consistently cell-mediated immunity, phagocytotic function, secretory antibody and cytokine production are affected (Chandra 1996). Worldwide, undernutrition is the commonest cause of immunodeficiency. Furthermore, malnutrition seems to have greater impact on bacterial than viral infections.

Another well known predisposing factor is diabetes mellitus. Diabetes mellitus leads to an increased susceptibility for bacterial infections. Gram positive bacteremia is more common in diabetic than in non diabetic patients (Leibovici et al. 1991). In the elderly patients diabetes, chronic obstructive lung disease and/or heart disease are associated with infectious complications, sepsis and death from septic shock (Rubio Felix et al. 1998). In a longitudinal cohort study it could be demonstrated that in patients with end-stage-renal disease infection is one of the most frequent causes of death, and prognosis of infectious diseases is worse in patients with diabetes (Powe et al. 1999). But even moderate renal insufficiency (serum creatinine < 3 mg/dl) indicates an increased risk. Patients with serum creatinine levels above 3 mg/dl have a nearly 2fold risk of death attributable to bacteremia (Shumuely et al. 2000).

Viral strategies to evade immune defenses affect immune competence, e.g. the production of glycoproteins by herpesviruses (herpes simplex viruses (HSV) and human cytomegalovirus (CMV)) interferes with complement activation and block the action of antiviral antibodies.

Seropositivity for CMV is associated with an increased risk for bacteremia and mortality, especially in transplant recipients, which affects survival after transplantation (Boston Center for Liver Transplantation CMVIG Study Group 1996). Throughout the AIDS epidemic, nosocomial and community acquired infections in the patient with HIV has presented an increasing problem. Opportunistic infections such as Pneumocystis carinii pneumonia, tuberculosis, CMV infections etc. are common, bacteremia and septic complications frequent (Laing et al. 1999).

There are many reports showing altered immune functions in patients after major trauma. Proinflammatory cytokines such as TNF-α and IL-6 have been found increased in most investigations, often showing an biphasic response. Depression of cellular immunity after major injury is frequently associated with subsequent infection (Faist et al. 1986). Trauma induced immuno-suppression may represent one of the most important predisposing factors for post-injury infections (Staphan 1987). The clinical consequences of these findings remain to be clarified. It is still unclear whether or not fractures of long bones should undergo primary internal fixation – despite of possible harms due to the altered immune function – or whether secondary osteosynthesis should be performed – with the risk of second hit phenomenon (Rixen et al. 2000).

Despite improvements in perioperative care and surgical techniques, severe infections are still major causes of postoperative mortality and morbidity in patients undergoing surgery. As stated for trauma also surgery alters the immune status of patients: Various investigations demonstrated altered cytokine profiles after major surgery. Serum levels of IL-6 increase within the first 24 hours (Ohzato et al. 1992), in contrast in vitro production of TNF-α and IL-1β of T-cells or monocytes decreases (Brune et al. 1999, Cabié et al. 1992). These alterations depend on the extent of surgery (Brune et al. 1999). In cancer patients *preoperatively* altered immune function has been detected (Saito et al. 1992) which may contribute to increased susceptibility to infection after surgery.

Postoperative Risk Factors

Chemo- and immunotherapeutic drugs obviously influence the immune status and everybody is aware of problems arising from those medications – but in clinical routine the effect of common drugs on the immune system is mostly neglected. ICU patients receive plenty of drugs possibly affecting inflammatory response. The following examples should draw attention to the influence of the all day ICU drugs on the immunological status of septic patients.

Treatment with corticosteroids is routine in many diseases. They have many important physiologic effects with substantial impact on the immune system. Apart from controlling an excessive immune response, there are several other potentially beneficial effects of corticosteroids in septic shock. However, whether (pre-)treatment with corticosteroids exhibits beneficial or deleterious effects is still discussed controversially (Meduri et al. 1998, Sprung 1998). A recently published systematic review concluded that preoperative methylprednisolone is not associated with significant increase in the incidence of adverse effects including infectious complications (Sauerland et al. 2000).

The release of bacterial cell wall components (LPS) can induce a substantial inflammatory response. Since the experiments of Richard Friedrich Pfeiffer in 1892 it is known that LPS can induce severe shock. β-lactam antibiotics (penicillin and cephalosporins) are rapidly bactericidal and enhance cell wall component release from both gram-negative and gram-positive bacteria. In a rabbit model of E. coli meningitis, cefotaxim therapy induced greater endotoxin release and brain oedema than did the protein synthesis inhibitor chloramphenicol

(Taber et al. 1987). Less has been reported so far about the antibiotic effect on gram-positive organisms. In a cell culture model of murine macrophages with pneumococci it has been demonstrated that oxacillin led to significantly higher inducible nitric oxide synthase and TNF-α accumulation than did clindamycin (Orman et al. 2000).

Catecholamines, which are part of the neurohumoral response to stress, show an inhibitory effect on the immune system. Catecholamine treatment reduces TNF-α and IL-1β production (van der Poll et al. 1996, Bergmann et al. 1999) and alters leukocyte numbers, neutrophil functions and lymphocyte subtypes (Burns et al. 1997). In patients with severe sepsis, endogenous catecholamines are elevated. The exogenously administered catecholamines can increase this level. Thus, endogenous and exogenous catecholamines may contribute to immunological anergy in sepsis.

1.3
Assessment of the Immunological Status

A variety of laboratory techniques are at hand to assess the immunological status of patients. Some analyses are done in clinical routine since many years (cell counts, C-reactive protein, skin tests). The following section will discuss parameters of possible prognostic value one may consider to determine in daily practice as well as some more sophisticated methods. The section is divided into 3 parts: the first part deals on cells, cellular functions and membrane receptors, followed by serum factors (cytokines and procalcitonin), the third part discusses in brief the possible importance of the genetic background.

Table 2. Laboratory parameters to assess the immunological status listed with regards to their availability and prognostic/clinical value

Parameter	Availability	Prognostic/clinical value
Cell counts	○	+
Cell subsets	○	+
Skin test	○	+
Phagocytosis in vivo	◇	+
Phagocytosis ex vivo	□	+
TNF-α	□	(+)
IL-1β	□	(+)
IL-4	□	(+)
IL-6	□	(+)
IL-10	□	(+)
CRP	○	–
Procalcitonin	○/□	+

Availability of laboratory parameters: ○ generally available in clinical routine, □ available in special settings, ◇ practicable in trials only; prognostic/clinical value: + clinical and experimental data, (+) Experimental data but clinical data controversial or missing, – no sufficient evidence.

1.3.1
Cell Counts, Cellular Functions and Membrane Receptors

Blood cell counts belong to daily clinical routine not only in ICU patients. Leuko-cytosis or leukopenia are very common in septic patients. Deviation of normal leukocyte counts is one out of four criteria for SIRS definition (Members of the American College of Chest Physicians/Society of Critical Care Medicine Consensus Conference Commitee 1992). White blood cell count on admission to ICU has shown to be an important risk factor for sepsis mortality (Knaus et al. 1993). However, in many septic patients leukocyte count remains unchanged.

Granulocytosis is a basic sign for bacterial infection, often associated with increased counts of juvenile forms which may also be the only sign. Monoclonal antibodies such as OKT3, OKT8, B1, etc. allow a detailed in vitro quantifica-tion of lymphocyte subpopulations. Clusters of differentiation (CD) have been defined for the most common monoclonal antibodies. $\alpha\beta$ T-cells can be subdivided by CD-markers into CD4 and CD8 cells. CD4+ T-cells recognize their specific antigens in association with MHC class II molecules, they mainly "help" or "induce" immune responses (TH). TH1-subsets are involved in several cytotoxic and local inflammatory reactions. TH2-subsets are more effec-tive stimulating B cells. Functional impairment and depletion of CD4+ T-cell subset over time is one of the leading pathophysiologic processes in patients with AIDS. But also malnutrition affects the cell-mediated immunity, indicated by a reduced number of CD4+ T-helper cells (Chandra 1983). TH1 immune response is down regulated after major surgery (Brune et al. 1999). The TH1/TH2 ratio in patients with severe sepsis is significantly lower than both non-septic controls and healthy subjects. The predominant TH2 mediated immune response may lead to fibroblast activation and immunosupression (Ferguson et al. 1999).

For clinical use some in vivo tests for immunofunction have been established. If skin test with recall antigens (such as tuberculin, tetanus antigen, etc.) are negative anergy of the cellular immune response has to be suspected. Negative skin-tests have been shown to be excellent preoperative predictors of postoper-ative septic complications (Meakins et al. 1980).

Phagocytosis can be determined in vivo by the clearance rate of radioactively labeled carbon or albumin beads or erythrocytes (Morgan and Soothill 1975, Low et al. 1985, Morgan and Steward 1976).

Measurement of phagocytosis can routinely be performed in vitro. A flow cytometric assay for phagocytosis of human blood monocytes has been devel-oped by Andoh et al. (Andoh et al. 1991) measuring the rate of cells internalizing fluorescent latex beads. Using a slightly modified method (measuring phago-cytosis of neutrophils) Hübel et al. demonstrated suppressed neutrophil func-tion as a risk factor for severe infection after chemotherapy (Hübel et al. 1999).

Superoxid production of neutrophil granulocytes, the premier event of the oxidative (respiratory) burst can also be determined using flow cytometry (Bass et al. 1983). Longitudinal analysis of neutrophil superoxide anion generation showed diminished oxidative burst in patients with septic shock in contrast to critically ill patients without sepsis right from day 0 of diagnosis.

Presentation of antigen by HLA class II molecules plays a critical role in specific immune response. Diminished expression of HLA-DR on monocyte surface is associated with infectious complications and postoperative sepsis (Wakefield et al. 1993). HLA-DR antigen expression on blood monocytes correlates with the incidence of surgical infection (Cheadle et al. 1991). But also after minor surgical interventions HLA-DR expression decreases (Carlei et al. 1999), which questions the clinical importance of HLA-DR suppression. Nevertheless, in a pilot study it was shown, that IFN-γ treatment of septic patients with downregulated monocytic HLA-DR expression resulted not only in recovery of monocyte function but also in clearance of sepsis in eight of nine patients (Doecke et al. 1997).

1.3.2
Serum Factors

Cytokines, a group of small proteins, are involved in a broad spectrum of biological functions and produced by a variety of cell types. Although originally believed that the primary role of cytokines was in immunologic homeostasis, it is now clear that certain cytokines also have profound effects on the intermediary metabolism, wound healing, and the cardiovascular system. The list of known cytokines in relation to sepsis is long and still expanding. Interleukins are of major interest for sepsis research since many years. ELISA kits allow measurement even routinely.

Primary responses to infectious insults have been studied in detail in animal models of endotoxemia. Responses to endotoxin challenge are mediated by pro-inflammatory cytokines such as tumor necrosis factor alpha (TNF-α) and interleukin-1 (IL-1). Pro-inflammatory mediators like interleukin-6 (IL-6) and interleukin-8 (IL-8) are induced by TNF-α and IL-1. A great variety of factors such as proteases, coagulation factors, kinins, eicosanoids, nitric oxide, and others have been described as mediators of immune functions. The following section will focus on the most established mediators (TNF-α, IL-1β, IL-6, IL-10).

TNF-α is secreted primarily by activated macrophages and is responsible for a variety of biological effects. It provides a potent stimulus for IL-1, IL-6 and IL-8 secretion. Systemic effects include fever, tachycardia, activation of neutrophils and complement. TNF-α is more increased in patients with Gram-negative than with Gram-positive infection. Patients without documented infection although fulfilling SIRS criteria have very low or even undetectable levels of TNF-α (Fisher et al. 1993). Non-survivors show significantly higher levels of TNF-α than survivors of septic shock (Martin et al. 1997). In trauma patients TNF-α-levels peak within the first hours. Due to the short half life of TNF-α elevation is variably found in studies. Moreover Riché and co-workers found increased levels of TNF-α associated with increased rather than decreased survival (Riché et al. 1996). In animal studies application of anti-TNF-antibodies resulted in a marked decrease of mortality (Cross et al. 1993, Hinshaw et al. 1990, Martin et al. 1993, Opal et al. 1991). Several studies investigated the effect of anti-TNF-strategies. However, they failed to demonstrate significant positive effects on mortality (Fisher et al. 1993, Bone 1996b, Cohen et al. 1996).

IL-1β is not consistently elevated in patients with sepsis or multiple organ failure (Pinsky et al. 1993) although endotoxemia induces release of both, IL-1β and interleukin-1 receptor antagonist (IL-1ra) (Granowiz et al. 1991). Based on positive results in animal studies IL1-ra has been used as therapeutic agent in several clinical trials. Although the open-label study showed a marked effect, the treatment effect was not statistically different in the two other studies (Fisher et al. 1994a, Fisher et al. 1994b, Opal et al. 1997).

IL-6 release is dramatically activated in patients with septic shock. Levels peak within the first day, going down over seven to ten days. Again, they are significantly higher in non-survivors than in survivors. In trauma patients IL-6 release is biphasic, peaking within the first hours and around day 8 to 10 (Martin et al. 1997, Hack et al. 1989). IL-6 levels correlate well with APACHE score and are by far more elevated in patients with shock. They may serve as a marker of severity (Damas 1992).

IL-4 and IL-10 are generally assumed to be anti-inflammatory cytokines. IL-4 is a potent T- and B-cell growth factor. During immune response it promotes expansion and differentiation of CD4+ TH2 cells, and expansion and differentiation of B-cells into immunoglobulin secreting cells. IL-4 lowers mortality rate in a murine model of LPS induced shock (Redmond et al. 1991, Giampetri 2000).

IL-10 which is secreted by various cell types, including lymphocytes and phagocytotic cells, has been shown to inhibit production of pro-inflammatory cytokines TNF-α, IL-1, and IL-8. Increased production of IL-10 after trauma has a negative impact on resistance to infection (Lyons et al. 1997). By interfering with the activation signals delivered by antigen-presenting cells, IL-10 acts indirectly on T-cells. It reduces the expression of class II major histocompatibility complex molecules at the monocyte surface. In a cecal ligation and puncture mouse model application of IL-10 prevented early cytokine release including TNF-α, IL-1β, and IL-6 (Rongione et al. 1997). It was also found to reduce endotoxin-induced mortality in mice (Ishida et al. 1993, Howard et al. 1993). However, these results could not be confirmed in a more clinically relevant mouse model (Remick et al. 1998).

The role of platelet activating factor (PAF) in the pathogenic mechanisms leading to sepsis has been extensively investigated. PAF is produced by numerous cell types including platelets, neutrophils, macrophages, endothelial and epithelial cells. Infusion of PAF produces a sepsis like state (Bessin et al. 1983). It has been found elevated in serum of septic patients in several but not all studies (Mathiak et al. 1997). Again clinical studies testing the efficacy of strategies directed against PAF in sepsis ended disappointing (BN 52021 Sepsis Study Group et al. 1994, Dhainaut et al. 1998).

CRP is known to be elevated early in the course of sepsis or septic shock and remains elevated throughout this period. Differences between survivors and non-nonsurvivors have not been detected (Wakefield et al. 1998). It therefore does not allow any prognostic differentiation.

Procalcitonin (PCT) is a prohormone which shows elevated plasma levels in severe bacterial, fungal, and parasitic infections as well as in sepsis and multi-organ failure. Autoimmune, allergic and viral diseases do not induce a rise in PCT. Its exact physiologic role is still unclear. PCT reflects the activity of systemic inflammatory reactions. In surgical ICU patients it has been shown that PCT mean levels of non-survivors of septic shock are significantly higher than those of survivors throughout the whole time course (Schröder et al. 1999). PCT was found to be closely related to postoperative complications with significantly elevated levels. In contrast IL-6 and CRP increase demonstrated no differences (Reith et al. 1998). This indicates that PCT may be a valuable parameter not only in the diagnosis of sepsis but also in the clinical course of the disease. Another more practical advantage of measuring PCT is that it is a stable molecule and cooling of plasma or serum probes is not required.

Although determining mediators as markers for the status of immune system in serum is a worthwhile approach, one has to be aware that infection often emerges locally. Circulating cytokines may be just the tip of the iceberg. Localised stimulation of leukocytes in organs such as the lung or Kupffer cells in the liver by infectious agents or mediators could induce local tissue injury and subsequent mortality without systemic dissemination of this cytokines. In animal studies it has been shown that intratracheal administration of E. coli results in a significant increase of TNF-α levels in BAL samples and concentrations in serum samples obtained form the aorta are significantly higher than those from arterial blood samples indicating that the lung is a major source of TNF-α. First clinical investigations on local cytokine concentrations could show that local cytokine profiles may be different from systemic levels. E.g. proinflammatory cytokines have been measured more elevated at local side in bronchoalveolar lavage of ICU patients with severe pneumonia (Montón et al. 1999, Mathiak et al. 2000) and in urine of patients with urosepsis (Olsazyna et al. 2000) than in serum. But we do not have a clear cut picture yet of the meaning of localized cell mediator interaction in terms of immunestatus and prognosis of the patients. Future investigations should help to understand the systemic importance of localised infection.

1.3.3
Genes

As discussed above sex differences play a critical role in sepsis development. However, little attention has been given to differences according to cytokine profiles yet. TNF-α, IL-6, PCT and IL-10 levels have been found to be significantly higher in men than in women (Schröder et al. 1998, Oberholzer et al. 2000) which may contribute to the worse outcome.

All genes encoding proteins involved in inflammatory responses are candidate genes to determine the human genetic background responsible for interindividual differences in systemic inflammatory response (Stüber et al. 1999). We are just in the beginning of unrevealing the codes for inflammatory proteins. Nevertheless, first investigations underline the potential role of a genetic background. A G-to-A-transition in the TNF-α gene has been associated with susceptibility to cerebral malaria (McGuire et al. 1994). A IL-1 genotype has been shown to be associated with outcome of meningococcal disease. Septic patients with a genomic polymorphic site of the restriction enzyme Ncol within the TNF locus have an increased mortality risk (Stuber et al. 1996). Polymorphism of the IL-1ra may contribute to susceptibility to sepsis (Fang et al. 1999). First protocols are on the way using gene therapy in infectious diseases (Santis et al. 1999). In the very near future microarray techniques will allow screening of patients for genetic deviation of many genes in parallel which may be associated with septic complications. Thus helping to identify genes and genetic defects which are involved in sepsis pathophysiology and in farer future identify patients as possible candidates for gene therapy.

1.4
Conclusions

Although the concept of cytokines as markers of the immunestatus is attractive, the difficulties and draw backs of this hypothesis have to be kept in mind. Definitive clinical or mechanistic conclusions about the role of cytokines and different cell types can not be drawn so far, since the frequency of cytokine detection and cell function measurements differ from series to series (Deitch 1993). Furthermore, most cytokines and cells have pleiotropic functions in the immune system. The understanding is complicated since the precise biological effect depends on the exact clinical circumstances. Depending on the cell type of the target cell and homeostatic cofactors a cytokine can act either as positive or negative signal. However, the first step has been done.

One of the major shortcomings of previous sepsis trials is that the identification of patients which may profit from a specific immunomodulatory therapy has not been taken under consideration. First trials considering this aspect are on their way. Hydrocortisone is given to patients included in an ongoing study of the French GER-INF-05 Group when they have a diminished ACTH response. First interim results are promising (Annane 2000).

A more precise understanding of the laboratory and clinical information of the immunstatus of patients will help giving the right (prophylactic or even therapeutic) drug to the right time for the right patient.

References

Andoh A, Fujiyama Y, Kitoh K, Hodohara K, Bamba T, Hosoda S (1991) Flow cytometric assay for phagocytosis of human monocytes mediated via Fc gamma-receptors and complement receptor CR1 (CD35). Cytometry 12: 677–686

Annane D (2000) Steroids for septic shock: the French randomised trial. Shock 13 (Suppl.): 160–161

Barclay GR (1995) Endogenous endotoxin-core antibody (EndoCAb) as a marker of endotoxin exposure and a prognostic indicator: a review. Prog Clin Biol Res 392: 263–272

Bartels H, Stein HJ, Siewert JR (1998) Preoperative risk analysis and postoperative mortality of oesophagectomy for resectable oesophageal cancer. Br J Surg 85: 840–844

Bass DA, Parce JW, Dechatelet LR, Szejda P, Seeds MC, Thomas M (1983) Flow cytometric studies of oxidative product formation by neutrophils: a graded response to membrane stimulation. J Immunol 130: 1910–1917

Bergmann M, Gornikiewicz A, Sautner T, Wladmann E, Weber T, Mittlböck M, Roth E, Függer R (1999) Attenuation of catecholamine-induced immunosuppression in whole blood from patients with sepsis. Shock 12: 421–427

Bessin P, Bonnet J, Apfel D, Soulard C, Desgroux L (1983) Acute circulating collapse caused by platelet activating factor (PAF acether) in dogs. Eur J Pharmacol 86: 403–440

Best GK, Scott DF, Kling M, Crowell WF, Kirkland JJ (1984) Enhanced susceptibility of male rabbits to infection with a toxic shock strain of Staphylococcus aureus. Infect Immun 46: 727–732

BN 52021 Sepsis Study Group, Dhainaut JF, Tenaillon A, Le Tulzo Y et al. (1994) Platelet-activating factor receptor antagonist BN 52021 in the treatment of severe sepsis: a randomized, double-blind, placebo-controlled, multicenter clinical trial. Crit Care Med 22: 1720–1728

Bone RC (1996) Sir Issac Newton, sepsis, SIRS, and CARS. Crit Care Med 24: 1125–1128

Bone RC (1996) Why sepsis trials fail. JAMA 276: 565–567

Boston Center for Liver Transplantation CMVIG Study Group, Falagas ME, Snydman DR, Griffith J, Werner BG (1996) Exposure to cytomegalovirus from the donated organ is a risk factor for bacteremia in orthotopic liver transplant recipients. Clin Infect Dis 23: 468–474

Brune IB, Wilke W, Hensler T, Holzmann B, Siewert JR (1999) Downregulation of T helper type 1 immune response and altered pro-inflammatory and anti-inflammatory T cell cytokine balance following conventional but not laparoscopic surgery. Am J Surg 177: 55–60

Burns AM, Keogan M, Donaldson M, Brown DL, Park GR (1997) Effects of inotropes on human leukocyte numbers, neutrophil function and lymphocyte subtypes. Br J Anaesth 78: 530–535

Cabié A, Fitting C, Farkas JC, Laurian C, Cornier JM, Carlet J, Cavaillon JM (1992) Influence of surgery on in-vitro cytokine production by human monocytes. Cytokine 4: 576–580

Carlei F, Schietroma M, Cianca G, Risetti A, Mattucci S, Ngome Enang G, Simi M (1999) Effects of laparoscopic and conventional (open) cholezystectomy on human leukocyted antigen-DR expression on peripheral blood monocytes: correlations with immunologic status. World J Surg 23: 18–22

Chandra RK (1983) Numerical and functional deficiency in T helper cells in protein energy malnutrition. Clin Exp Immunol 51: 123–132

Chandra RK (1996) Nutrition, immunity and infection. Proc Natl Acad Sci USA 93: 14304–14307

Cheadle WG, Hershman MJ, Wellhausen SR, Polk HC (1991) HLA-DR antigen expression on peripheral blood immunocytes correlates with surgical infection. Am J Surg 161: 639–646

Cohen J, Carlet H, Intersept Study Group (1996) INTERSEPT: An international, multicenter, placebo-controlled trial of monoclonal antibody to human tumor necrosis factor-α in patients with sepsis. Crit Care Med 24: 1431–1440

Cross AS, Opal SM, Palardy JE, Bodmer MW, Sadoff JC (1993) The efficacy of combination immunotherapy in experimental Pseudomonas sepsis. J Infect Dis 167: 112–118

Damas P, Ledoux D, Nys M, Vrindts Y, De Groote D, Franchimont P, Lamy M (1992) Cytokine serum level during severe sepsis in human: IL-6 as a marker of severitiy. Ann Surg 215: 356–362

Deitch EA (1993) Cytokines yes, cytokines no, cytokines maybe? Crit Care Med 21: 817–819

Dhainaut JFA, Tenaillon A, Hemmer M, Damas P, Le Tulzo Y, Radermacher P, Schaller MD, Sollet JP, Wolff M, Holzapfel L, Zeni F, Vedrinne JM, de Vathaire F, Gourlay ML, Duinot P, Mira JP, BN 52021 Sepsis Investigator Group (1998) Confirmatory platelet-activating factor receptor antagonist trial in patients with severe Gram-negative bacterial sepsis: a phase III, randomized, double-blind, placebo-controlled, multicenter trial. Crit Care Med 26: 1963–1971

Doecke WD, Randow F, Syrbe U, Krausch D, Asadullah K, Reinke P, Volk HD, Kox W (1997) Monocyte deactivation in septic patients: restoration by IFN-gamma treatment. Nat Med 3: 678–681

Faist E, Kupper T, Baker CC, Chaudry IH, Dwyer J, Bauer AE (1986) Depression of cellular immunity after major injury: its association with post traumatic complications and its reversal with immunomodulation. Arch Surg 121: 1000–1005

Fang XM, Schröder S, Hoeft A, Stüber F (1999) Comparison of two polymorphisms of the interleukin-1 gene family: interleukin-1 receptor antagonist polymorphism contributes to susceptibility to severe sepsis. Crit Care Med 27: 1330–1334

Ferguson NR, Galley HF, Webster NR (1999) T helper cell subset ratios in patients with severe sepsis. Intensive Care Med 25: 106–109

Fisher CJ, Opal SM, Dhainaut JF, Stephens S, Zimmerman JL, Nightingale P, Harris SJ, Schein RM, Panacek EA, Vincent JL, Foulke GE, Warren EL, Garrard C, Park G, Bodmer MW, Cohen J, van der Linden C, Cross AS, Sadoff JC, the CB0006 Sepsis Syndrome Study Group (1993) Influence of an anti-tumor necrosis factor monoclonal antibody on cytokine levels in patients with sepsis. Crit Care Med 21: 318–327

Fisher CJ, Dhainaut JF, Opal SM, Pribble JP, Balk RA, Slotman GJ, Iberti TJ, Rackow EC, Shapiro MJ, Greenman RL et al. (1994) Recombinant human interleukin 1 receptor antagonist in the treatment of patients with sepsis syndrome. Results from a randomized, double-blind, placebo-controlled trial. Phase III rhIL-1ra Sepsis Syndrome Study Group. JAMA 23: 1836–1843

Fisher CJ, Slotman GJ, Opal SM, Pribble JP, Bone RC, Emmanuel G, Ng D, Bloedow DC, Catalano MA, IL-1 RA Sepsis Syndrome Study Group T (1994) Initial evaluation of human recombinant interleukin-1 receptor antagonist in the treatment of sepsis syndrome: a randomized, open-label, placebo-controlled multicenter trial. Crit Care Med 22: 12–21

Giampietri A, Grohmann U, Vacca C, Fioretti MC, Pucetti P, Campanile F (2000) Dual effect of IL-4 on resistance to systemic gram-negative infection and production of TNF-alpha. Cytokine 12: 417–421

Granowiz EV, Santos AA, Poutsiaka DD, Cannon JG, Wilmore DW, Wolff SM, Dinarello CA (1991) Production of interleukin-1-receptor antagonist during experimental endotoxemia. Lancet 338: 1423–1424

Hack CE, De Groot ER, Felt-Bersma RJF, Nuijens JH, van Schijndel RJMS, Eerenberg-Belmer AJM, TLG, Aarden LA (1989) Increased plasma levels of interleukin-6 in sepsis. Blood 74: 1704–1710

Hinshaw LB, Olson PT, Chang AC, Lee PA, Taylor FB, Murray CK, Peer GT, Emerson TE, Passey RB, Kuo GC (1990) Survival of primates in LD100 septic shock following therapy with antibody to tumor necrosis factor (TNF alpha). Circ Shock 30: 279–292

Howard M, Muchamuel T, Andrade S, Menon S (1993) Interleukin 10 protects mice from lethal endotoxemia. J Exp Med 177: 1205–1208

Hübel K, Hegener K, Schnell R, Mansmann G, Oberhäuser F, Staib P, Diehl V, Engert A (1999) Suppressed neutrophil function as a risk factor for severe infection after cytotoxic chemotherapy in patients with acute nonlymphcytic leukemia. Ann Hematol 78: 37–77

Ishida H, Hastings R, Thompson-Snipes L, Howard M (1993) Modified immunological status of anti-IL-10 treated mice. Cell Immunol 148: 371–384

Kawakami K, Kadota J, Iida K, Shirai R, Abe K, Kohno S (1999) Reduced immune function and malnutrition in the elderly. Tholku J Exp Med 187: 157–171

Knaus WA, Harrell FE, Fisher CF, Wagner DP, Opal SM, Sadoff JC, Draper EA, Walawander CA, Conboy K, Grasela TH (1993) The clinical evaluation of new drugs for sepsis. JAMA 270: 1233–1241

Laing RB (1999) Nosocomial infections in patients with HIV disease. J Hosp Infect 43: 179–185

Leibovici L, Samra Z, Konisberger H, Kalter-Leibovici O, Pitlik SD, Drucker M (1991) Bacteriemia in adult diabetic patients. Diabetes Care 14: 89–94

Lesuord B., Mazari L (1999) Nutrition and immunity in the elderly. Proc Nutr Soc 58: 685–695

Low A, Hotze A, Krapf F, Schranz W, Manger BJ, Mahlstedt J, Wolf F, Kalden JR (1985) The nonspecific clearance function of the reticuloendothelial system in patients with immune complex mediated diseases before and after therapeutic plasmapheresis. Rheumatol Int 5: 69–72

Lyons A, Kelly JL, Rodrcik ML, Mannick JA, Lederer JA (1997) Major injury induces increased production of interleukin-10 by cells of the immune system with a negative impact on resistance to infection. Ann Surg 226: 450–460

Majetschak M, Christensen B, Obertacke U, Waydhas C, Schindler AE, Nast-Kolb D, Schade FU (2000) Sex differences in posttraumatic cytokine release of endotoxin-stimulated whole blood: relationship to the development of severe sepsis. J Trauma 48: 832–840

Martin RA, Silva AT, Cohen J (1993) Effect of anti TNF-α treatment in an antibiotic treated murine model of shock due to Streptococcus pyogenes. FEMS Microbiol Lett 110: 175–178

Martin C, Boisson C, Haccoun M, Thomachot L, Mege JL (1997) Patterns of cytokine evolution (tumor necrosis factor-α and interleukin-6) after septic shock, hemorrhagic shock, and severe trauma. Crit Care Med 25: 1813–1819

Mathiak G, Szwecyk D, Abdullah F, Ovadia P, Rabinovici R (1997) Platelet-activating factor (PAF) in experimental and clinical sepsis. Shock 7: 391–404

Mathiak G, Luebke T, Herzmann T, Grass G, Boehm SA, Mueller C, Beckurts KTE, Helling HJ, Hoelscher AH (2000) Putative role for locally produced chemokines in early human sepsis In: Faist E. 5th world congress on trauma, shock, inflammation and sepsis: pathophysiology, immune consequences and therapy. Bologna: Monduzzi Editore, 39–42

McGuire W, Hill AV, Allsopp CE, Greenwood BM, Kwiatkowski D (1994) TNF-alpha promoter region associated with susceptibility to cerebral malaria. Nature 371: 508–510

Meakins JL, Pietsch JB, Christou NV, Maclean LD (1980) Predicting surgical infection before the operation. World J Surg 4: 439–450

Meduri GU, Kanangat S (1998) Glucocorticoid treatment of sepsis and acute respiratory distress syndrome: time for a critical reappraisal. Crit Care Med 26: 630–633

Members of the American College of Chest Physicians/Society of Critical Care Medicine Consensus Conference Commitee (1992) American College of Chest Physician/Society of Critical Care Medicine Consensus Conference: definitions for sepsis and organ failure and guidelines for the use of innovative therapies in sepsis. Crit Care Med 20: 864–874

Montón C, Torres A, El-Ebiary M, Filella X, Xaubet A, de la Bellacasa JP (1999) Cytokine expression in severe pneumonia: a bronchoalveolar lavage study. Crit Care Med 27: 1745–1753

Morgan AG, Soothill JF (1975) Measurement of the clearance function of macrophages with [125]J-labeled polyvinyl pyrrolidone. Clin Exp Immunol 20: 489–496

Morgan AG, Steward MW (1976) Macrophage clearance function and immune complex disease in New Zealand Black/White F1 hybrid mice. Clin Exp Immunol 26: 133–136

Neugebauer E, Rixen D, Raum M, Schäfer U (1998) Thirty years of anti-mediator treatment in sepsis and septic-shock what have we learned? Langenbecks Arch Surg 383: 26–34

Oberholzer A, Kerel M, Zellweger R, Steckholzer U, Trentz O, Ertel W (2000) Incidence of septic complications and multiple organ failure in severely injured patients is sex specific. J Trauma 48: 932–937

Ohzato H, Yoshizaki K, Nishimoto N, Ogata A, Tagoh H, Monden M, Gotoh M, Kishimoto T, Mori T (1992) Interleukin-6 as a new indicator of inflammatory status: detection of serum levels of interleukin-6 and C-reactive protein after surgery. Surgery 111: 201–209

Olsazyna DP, Opal SM, Prins JM, Horn DL, Speelman P, van Deventer SJH, van der Poll T (2000) Chemotactic activity of CXC chemokines interleukin-8, growth-related oncogene-alpha, and epithelial cell-derived neutrophil-activating protein-78 in urine of patients with urosepsis. J Infect Dis 182: 1731–1737

Opal SM, Cross AS, Sadoff JC, Collins HH, Kelly NM, Victor GH, Palardy JE, Bodmer MW (1991) Efficacy of antilipopolysaccharide and anti-tumor necrosis factor monoclonal antibodies in a neutropenic rat model of Pseudomonas sepsis. J Clin Invest 88: 885–890

Opal SM, Fisher CJ, Dhainaut JFA, Vincent JL, Brase R, Lowry SF, Sadoff JC, Slotman GJ, Levy H, Balk RA, Shelly MP, Pribble JP, LaBrecque JF, Lookabaugh J, Donovan H, Dubin H, Baughman R, Norman J, DeMaria E, Matzel K, Abraham E, Seneff M (1997) Interleukin-1 Receptor Antagonist Sepsis Investigator Group. Confirmatory interleukin-1 receptor antagonist trial in severe sepsis: a phase III, randomized, double-blind, placebo-controlled, multicenter trial. Crit Care Med 25: 1115–1124

Orman KL, English BK (2000) Effects of antibiotic class on the macrophage inflammatory response to streptococcus pneumonia. J Infect Dis 182: 1561–1565

Pinsky MR, Vincent JL, Deviere J, Alegre M, Kahn RJ, Dupont E (1993) Serum cytokine levels in human septic shock: relation to multiple-system organ failure and mortality. Chest 103: 565–575

Pittet D, Thievent B, Wenzel RP, Li N, Gurman G, SPM (1993) Importance of pre-existing co-morbidities for prognosis of septicemia in critically ill patients. Intensive Care Med 19: 265–272

Powe NR, Jaar B, Furth SL, Hermann J, Briggs W (1999) Septicemia in dialysis patients: incidence, risk factors, and prognosis. Kidney Int 55: 1081–1090

Redmond HP, Chavin KD, Bromberg JS, Daly JM (1991) Inhibition of macrophage-activating cytokines is beneficial in the acute septic response. Ann Surg 214: 502–509

Reith HB, Mittelkötter U, Debus ES, Küssner C, Thiede A (1998) Procalcitonin in early detection of postoperative complications. Dig Surg 15: 260–265

Remick DG, Garg SJ, Newcomb DE, Wollenberg G, Huie TK, Bolgos GL (1998) Exogenous interleukin-10 fails to decrease the mortality or morbidity of sepsis. Crit Care Med 26: 895–904

Riché F, Panis Y, Lasiné MJ, Birard C, Cholley B, Bernard-Poenaru O, Graulet AMGJVP (1996) High tumor necrosis factor serum level is associated with increased survival in patients with abdominal septic shock: a prospective study in 59 patients. Surgery 120: 801–807

Rixen D, Bouillon B, Sauerland S, Grass G, Neugebauer E (2000) In search of the optimal time point for long-bone fracture surgery in multiple trauma patients with brain injury – where is the evidence? Restor Neurol Neurosci 16: 265–266

Rongione AJ, Kusske AM, Ashley SW, Reber HA, McFadden DW (1997) Interleukin-10 prevents early cytokine release in severe intraabdominal infection and sepsis. J Surg Res 70: 107–112

Rubio Felix S, Aznar Munoz R, Martin Algora I, Egido Murciano M, Ferrero Cancer M, Mairal Claver P, Rezusta Lopez A (1998) Bactermemia in the elderly: associated and prognostic factors. Rev Clin Esp 198: 7–10

Saito T, Shigemitsu Y, Kinoshita T, Shimoda K, Miyahara M, Kobayashi M (1992) Impaired neutrophil bactericidal activity correlates with the infection occuring after surgery for esophageal cancer. J Surg Oncol 51: 159–163

Santis G, Evans TW (1999) Molecular biology for the critical care physician. Part II: where are we now? Crit Care Med 27: 997–1003

Sauerland S, Nagelschmidt M, Mallmann P, Neugebauer EAM (2000) Risks and benefits of preoperative high dose methylprednisolone in surgical patients: a systematic review. Drug Saf 5: 449–461

Schröder J, Kahlke V, Staubach KH, Zabel P, Stüber F (1998) Gender differences in human sepsis. Arch Surg 133: 1200–1205

Schröder J, Staubach KH,ZP, Stüber F, Kremer B (1999) Procalcitonin as a marker of severity in septic shock. Langenbecks Arch Surg 384: 33–38

Shumuely H, Pitlik S, Drucker M, Samra Z, Konisberger H, Leibovici L (2000) Prediction of mortality in patients with bacteremia: the importance of pre-existing renal insufficiency. Ren Fail 22: 99–108

Spijkstra JJ, Girbes ARJ (2000) The continuing story of corticosteroids in the treatment of septic shock. Intensive Care Med 26: 496–500

Sprung CL (1998) Corticosteroids in septic shock: resurrection of the last rites? Crit Care Med 26: 627–630

Staphan RNKTS, Qeha AS, Baue AE, Chaudry IH (1987) Hemorrhage without tissue trauma produces immunosuppresion and enhances susceptability to sepsis. Arch Surg 122: 62–68

Stüber F (1999) Human responses to endotoxin: role of the genetic background In: Brade H, Opal SM, Vogel SN, Morrison DC. Endotoxin in health and disease. New York: Marcel Decker, 877–885

Stuber F, Petersen M, Bokelmann F, Schade U (1996) A genomic polymorphism within the tumor necrosis factor locus influences plasma tumor necrosis factor-alpha concentrations and outcome of patients with severe sepsis. Crit Care Med 24: 381–384

Taber MG, Shibl AM, Hackbarth CJ, Larrcik JW, Sande MA (1987) Antibiotic therapy, endotoxin concentration in cerebrospinal fluid, and brain edema in experimental Escherichia coli meningitis in rabbits. J Infect Dis 156: 456–462

Tang E, Tang G, Berne TV (1993) Prognostic indicators in fungemia of the surgical patient. Arch Surg 128: 759–762

van der Poll T, Coyle SM, Barbosa K, Braxton CC, Lowry SF (1996) Epinephrine inhibits tumor necrosis factor alpha and potentiates interleukin-10 production during human endotemia. J Clin Invest 97: 713–719

Wakefield CH, Carey PD, Foulds S, Monson JRT, Guillou PJ (1993) Changes in major histocompatibility complex class II expression immunocytes and T-cells of patients developing infection after surgery. Br J Surg 80: 205–209

Wakefield CH, Barclay GR, Fearon KCH, Goldie AS, Ross JA, Grant IS, Ramsay G, Howie JC (1998) Proinflammatory mediator activity, endogenous antagonists and the systemic inflammatory response in intra-abdominal sepsis. Br J Surg 85: 818–825

Wichmann MW, Inthorn D, Schildberg FW (1998) Incidence and mortality of severe sepsis in surgical intensive care-influence of gender on disease process and out-come. Shock 10 (Suppl.): 3

Zellweger R, Wichmann MW, Ayala A, Stein S, DeMaso CM, Chaudry IH (1997) Females in proestrus state maintain splenic immune functions and tolerate sepsis better than males. Crit Care Med 25: 106–110

Markers of Inflammation for Prognosis and Control of Therapeutic Success in Patients with Abdominal Sepsis – Options for Using Adjuvant Intravenous Immunoglobulins

H. B. REITH and U. MITTELKÖTTER

2.1
Introduction

Sepsis is first of all a clinical diagnosis and is based on objective clinical data according to the ACCP/SCCM-definitions from 1991, which defined sepsis as a situation with an identified or obvious infection and the criteria of systemic inflammatory response syndrome (SIRS). These criteria are temperature more than 38.4 °C or less than 36.0 °C, tachycardia of more than 90 heartbeats/minute, tachypnoea of more than 20 breaths/minute or the need for artificial ventilation and a leukocyte count of more than 12000/µl or less than 4000/µl.

Up to now there is no correlation between microbiological diagnostic procedures and results and the clinical sign of sepsis. During the period of one year (may 1997 – may 1998) we evaluated 105 patients (out of 406 patients) which were admitted into the surgical ICU with a primary infection and/or sepsis. A community aquired infection was found in 29% of the cases with a positive microbiological finding in 45%, 71% of these patients have had a nosocomial aquired infection with a positive microbiological finding in 56%.

The initial idea to establish definitions for SIRS and sepsis was fabulous, however, the criticism of this definitions started at the very time as their introduction.

One criticism is, that for example if someone chases a dog, he or she will show enough of the above mentioned clinical signs to meet the criteria for SIRS. The difference in our opinion is, that while this type of "SIRS" resolves within a few minutes, a patient on an ICU has SIRS for a longer period of time leading to either restitution or development of sepsis.

2.2
Prognostic Approaches

2.2.1
Scoring Systems

The work of Rangel-Frausto and coworkers of 1995 demonstrates the correlations (Fig. 1) between mortality and severity of SIRS and sepsis (Rangel-Frausto et al. 1995). Although these definitions detecting patients with inflammation and

Fig. 1. Mortality rate of systemic inflammatory response syndrome (SIRS) and sepsis in a prospective trial with 2527 patients independent from culture positive or negative findings (adapted from 1)

Criteria	Mortality rate (%)
no SIRS	3
SIRS (2 criteria)	7
SIRS (3 criteria)	10
SIRS (4 criteria)	17
Sepsis	16
severe sepsis	20
septic shock	46

sepsis present a wide range, there is a strong correlation to mortality rates and they are useful for prognostic evaluation. On the other hand, negative findings of the SIRS-criteria may be found in patients after trauma and non-infective pancreatitis, and sometimes the parameters are quite normal compared to the clinical impact of a septic focus and for example the need of a surgical therapy.

Different scoring systems and other measurements have been developed to monitor the septic course, but they have limitations in predicting individual outcome. Evaluations have been carried out for scores like APACHE II, MOF-Score from Goris and SOFA-Score (Le Gall JR et al. 1993; Reist et al. 1996; Bein and Unertl 1993).

2.2.2
CRP

C-reactive protein (CRP) is a well known marker of infective processes. CRP is an acute-phase protein, produced in hepatocytes following stimulation by interleukin-6 (Il-6). An increase of CRP is also found after trauma, surgery, in chronic infectious diseases and sometimes in patients with malignancies. The period of time to response is between 24 and 48 hours. However, an increase or decrease of CRP is not always correlated with the development or disappearing of an infectious focus. CRP also failed to be of immediate diagnostic and prognostic help due to the delay of production and the duration of increased serum concentrations (Heney et al. 1992; Heuer et al.: 1991; Rosman et al. 1993). CRP is triggered by nearly all inflammatory and infectious processes. Postoperatively surgical patients show a CRP-elevation within two days evoked by surgery itself. CRP normally decreases with a half-life time of 24 hours. Depending on the peak level, postoperative patients may have elevated CRP-values for up to 8 days.

Although during infections CRP also increases and thus could be a useful marker at an early stage to determine the severity of infection in clinical studies, with repeated infective stimuli, however, CRP is not adequately re-stimulated.

2.3
The Immune System

The immune system is an "organ-like" system with outstanding functions for the whole organism. Each organ system in the body is generating a variety of markers and parameters to allow a correct diagnosis of functional disorders. Since these parameters need more or less invasive monitoring, researchers concentrate on only one of them. But we have to take into account, that one single marker of the organic function gives information on only one part of the organic function. The same situation is found in the immune system: measuring one single marker of course can not reflect the whole function of the system.

2.3.1
Pro- and Antiinflammatory Reactants

As proposed in a lot of studies, pro- and antiinflammatory reactions occur simultaneously. Therefore it is necessary to monitor both the pro- and the anti-inflammatory reactions.

The proinflammatory cytokines (f.e. TNF-α, Il-6) are early mediators of inflammation and infection response. Postoperative patients also show a release of these mediators and as far as we know today, the type of operation determines the median values of Il-6 production. In patients with infections the Il-6 concentrations are higher with values of more than 1000 pg/mL when these patients suffer from sepsis and organ dysfunction disorders. Although this difference is acceptable to decide on treatment regimes, we do not know exactly whether this is a prognostic tool or not. A multicenter assessment for the outcome of septic patients with Il-6 values of more than 1000 pg/mL is still ongoing (SELECT-1-study). The results may help to clarify the question: can cytokine concentrations be used as prognostic tools for patients prone to septic complications?

But it may be assumed that due to the short half-life of most of the inter-leukins an interpretation of cytokine plasma levels will still be difficult.

The antiinflammatory reaction is an immunosuppressive event. Interleukin-10 (Il-10) is one of the prominent promotors of immunosuppression. The release of Il-10 is stimulated directly by the central-nervous system ("stress"), the immune system and also by drugs (catecholamines and others). The grade of this suppression can be measured by Il-10 concentrations in the plasma as well as by the expression of human leucocyte antigens (HLA) on the surface of monocytes. Even better is the measurement of HLA-DR expression.

2.3.2
HLA-DR Expression on Monocytes

The expression of antigens (f.e. HLA-DR) on monocytes plays an important role for an adequate response of the immune system. The HLA-DR expression is an alternative, more or less a surrogate parameter for the measurement of immuno-suppression, f.e. for reduced leukocyte response and for release of mediators as a feed-back mechanism to modulate cytokine reactions. There are several reports about the reduction of this expression in patients after trauma, shock and sepsis (Döcke et al. 1997). This reduction has a prognostic relevance in the follow-up of an infection and seems to be of prognostic relevance in septic diseases, as the group of Volk and coworkers has demonstrated (Döcke et al. 1997).

They showed that with a HLA-DR expression below 30% within 5 days, the survival rate was 12%. In contrast in septic patients having either normal values, a shorter period of immunosuppression or only one or two episodes of reduced HLA-DR expression values the survival rate was 88%.

In patients with abdominal sepsis due to peritonitis this kind of monitoring is a new approach in the control of the immune system.

2.3.3
The Value of Determining Monocytic HLA-DR Expression in Clinical Practice

We used the two-colour-fluorescence activated cell sorter (FACS) method to identify monocytes with monoclonal antibodies (CD 14) and to measure the

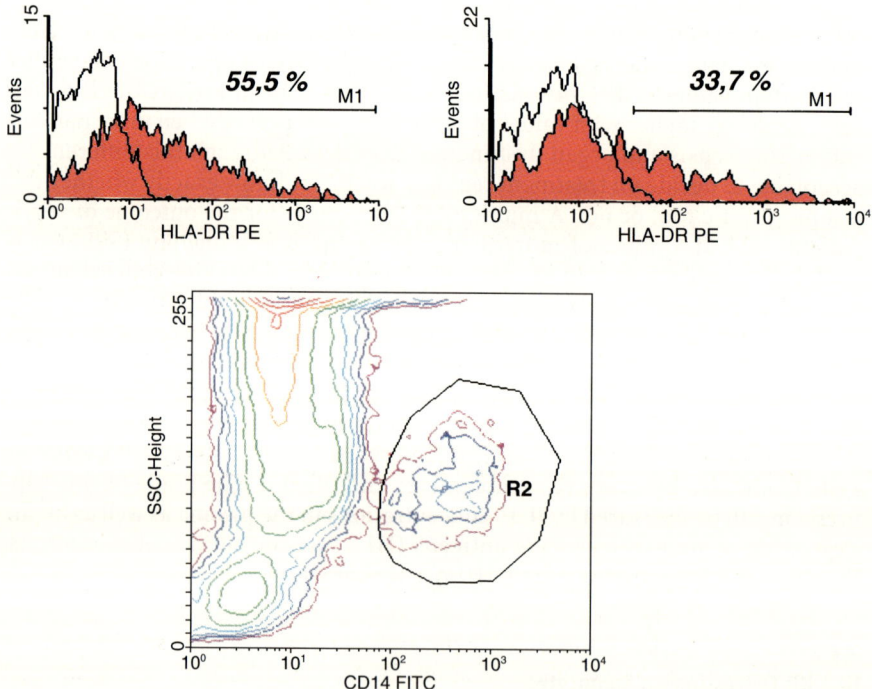

Fig. 2. HLA-DR expression on CD 14 positive monocytes marked with R2 (in the lower part). The area under curve (AUC) of the HLA-DR expression is determined as area minus the area of baseline fluorescence (55,5%, left side – black line) and isotype control (33,7%, right side – black line). The AUC is different depending on the used techniques of measurement in the same patient with a severe sepsis due to peritonitis

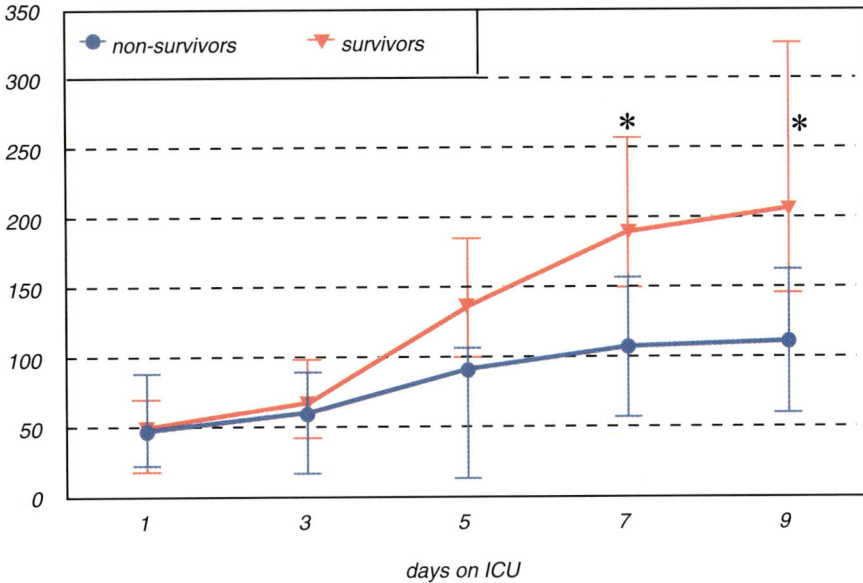

Fig. 3. Results of HLA-DR expression in survivors and non-survivors in an ICU follow-up, results in MFI/MFI-autofluorescence quotient. There is a statistically significant difference for days 7 and 9 (Mann-Whitney-U-Test, p < 0.05)

HLA-DR expression (both antibodies from Beckman-Coulter, Krefeld, Germany). We used the FACS-scan of Becton & Dickinson, Heidelberg, Germany. The identification was carried out with the forward and sideward scatter (Fig. 2). The mean channel fluorescence intensity (MFI) is a reliable parameter for sequential measurements. Figure 3 shows two groups of patients suffering from diffuse peritonitis in the situation of immunosuppression according to a MFI/MFI autofluorescence-quotient below 120. During follow-up the groups differ in their outcome in survivors, who recover within a few days and for non-survivors, who remain in a bad condition over the whole period. HLA-DR expression is therefore of prognostic value according to the results of the Volk group. However, the problem of technique standardisation for FACS-scan is still unsolved.

2.3.4
Use of Monocytic HLA-DR Expression for Patient Selection

One aim for the future is the focus on prevention of infective and septic episodes and to avoid postoperative complications like organ failure. In a first attempt we tried to find out the immunological reactivity in patients with oncological procedures, like esophageal cancer and gastric cancer resection. We compared those patients to a group of laparoscopic fundoplicatio operations. The group of patients with infective or septic complications had a reduced HLA-DR expression in the preoperative period already (Fig. 4). The results are of high statistical

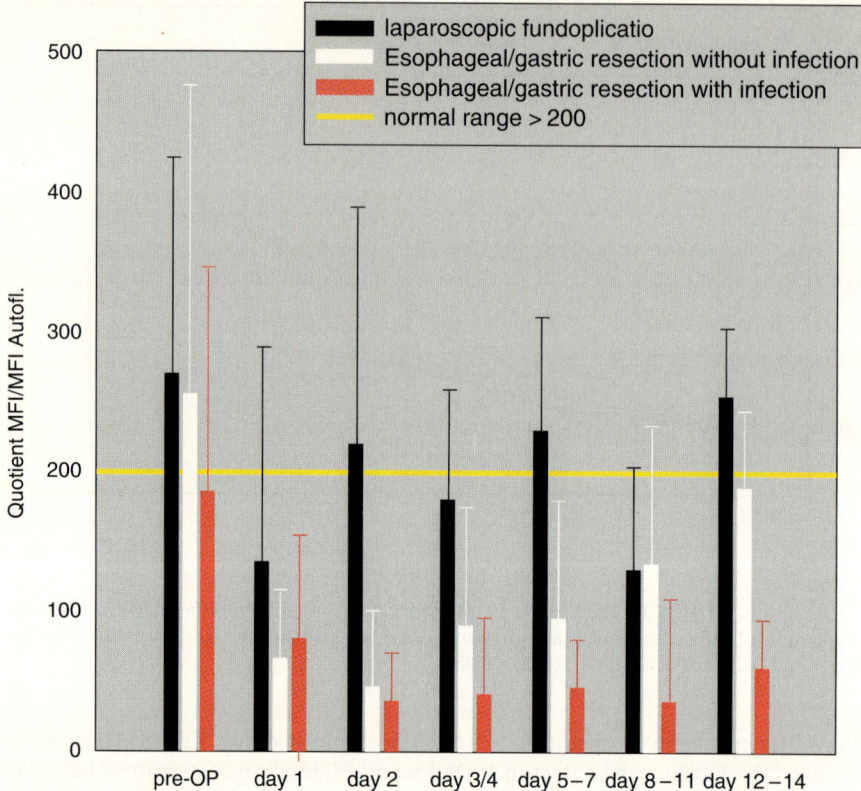

Fig. 4. Results of HLA-DR expression on monocytes in elective surgery. Risk stratification by preoperative measurement to identify groups on risk for infective or septic complication. An interesting new method for sepsis prevention. The results are statistically significant for pre-operative day, day 3–4, day 5–7, day 8–11 and day 12–14 (p < 0.001)

significance. In consequence of these results a preoperative routine measurement of HLA-DR expression was established. Furthermore we are planning a clinical trial to prove the concept of immune-stimulating procedures preoperatively.

2.4
Procalcitonin

The cascade of cytokine secretion induced by systemic infection, may damage the tight junctions between the inner and outer parts of the cell membranes of neuroendocrine cells. Apical cell membranes usually secrete mature hormones, and basolateral membranes secrete incompletely processed prohormones. The loss of polarity of an epithelial cell converts its entire cell membrane into a baso-lateral membrane. Consequently the Golgi apparatus receives the message to produce predominantly non-processed or incompletely processed prohormones, like the procalcitonin. Procalcitonin is a 116 amino acid peptide that contains calcitonin (a 32 amino acid part of the prohormone) and katacalcin (another determined part of the prohormone). The katacalcin sequence is different in PCT I for inflammatory and infectious reactions and PCT II in thyroid cells. Now we are able to demonstrate that prohormones like the PCT are released after an inflammatory stimulus (trauma, operation), stress and infection. Monocytes will have an increase in m-RNA coding for PCT, however they need a cell contact to release PCT into the blood stream (Assiot et al. 1993; Becker et al. 1981).

2.4.1
PCT in a Prospective Study – Own Results

In a prospective study we measured procalcitonin in 246 patients with septic syndrome or infections after abdominal surgery due to peritonitis. Peritonitis was suspected as follows: local inflammation of the peritoneum, exsudate, GI-tract perforation or ileus (Table 1). We defined sepsis according to Bone's criteria (Bone 1991). Criteria for inclusion into the study were clinical and objective diagnoses of sepsis and an APACHE II-score of 15 points or more. All patients required artificial ventilation. A votum of the local ethic committee was confirmed. Exclusion criteria were pregnancy, breast feeding, treatment with any other investigational drug, progressive fatal disease, onset of pancreatitis and patients with planned relaparotomies.

TNF-α, Il-6, neopterin, CRP, and other standard laboratory variables were also measured to validate the procalcitonin values. TNF-α, IL-6, and neopterin were analysed with a specific enzyme-linked immunosorbent assay (ELISA, Biosource Diagnostics, Solingen, Germany or B.R.A.H.M.S Diagnostica GmbH, Hennigsdorf, Germany). CRP-concentrations were analysed with a nephelometric assay (Dade Behring Diagnostics, Marburg, Germany). Concentrations of pro-

Table 1. Diagnosis in patients developing abdominal infection and SIRS

Diagnosis	Total No	No (%) Deaths
Pancreatitis	24	5 (21)
Colon perforation	99	16 (16)
Postoperative peritonitis		
* Anastomotic leakage	33	15 (45)
* Abscess	26	4 (15)
Biliary peritonitis	4	1 (25)
Traumatic peritonitis	19	3 (16)
Mesenterial infarction	40	14 (35)
Others	1	1 (100)
Total	246	59 (24)

calcitonin were measured with a specific, ultrasensitive, immunoluminometric assay (LUMItest® PCT assay, B.R.A.H.M.S Diagnostica, Hennigsdorf, Germany).

The 246 patients were assessed daily during their stay on the intensive care unit (ICU) to document the course of the infection until death or discharge. The first clinical classification was initially made using the APACHE II score and the follow up was monitored by the multiple organ failure (MOF)-score (Goris RJA et al. 1985).

2.4.2
Results

Patients with peritonitis, pancreatitis and sepsis always had increased concentrations of procalcitonin. A decrease of the procalcitonin concentration correlated with clinical improvement of infection and sepsis, and was found in all surviving patients. The 59 patients who died had initial procalcitonin values of 4.2 ± 1.3 ng/ml rising to a mean of 13.8 ± 8.9 ng/ml on day 1, 13.0 ± 7.5 ng/ml on day 4 and 13.2 ± 5.8 ng/ml at the time of death. The 187 patients who survived infection or sepsis, had an initial concentration of 2.1 ± 0.7 ng/ml, 4.9 ± 2.8 ng/ml on day 1, 4.8 ± 3.1 ng/ml on day 4, followed by a reduction to the mean reference range of 0.4 ± 0.1 ng/ml. Compared to the values for CRP, PCT showed significant differences between survivors and patients who died ($p < 0.05$ on days 1 and 4 and at the endpoint); whereas CRP did not.

Of particular interest were results from patients who developed infection or sepsis during the observation period. In these cases PCT and TNF increased at the same time preceding the rise of IL-6. There was a good correlation with the MOF score ($r = 0.83$).

The APACHE II score for patients who died (20.9 ± 3.3 points) and those who survived (20.1 ± 3.6 points) was initially similar. The MOF score for those who died ranged from 5 – 12 points (mean 9.6 ± 3.7 points) and for the survivors from 0 – 9 (mean 2.8 ± 1.8 points). The mortality (59/246) was 24% (Reith et al. 2000)

The prognostic value of procalcitonin has been convincingly verified by meta-analysis (Beier 1994). Our results are similar to other studies on burns and adult respiratory distress syndrome, which reported that an increase or a constant high level in procalcitonin concentrations predicted a lethal outcome (Huttemeier et al. 1993; Joyce et al. 1990; Mimos et al. 1998; Brunkhorst et al. 1992; Nylen et al. 1992) (the sensitivity was 84% and the specificity 91%).

2.5
Other Mediators

Of course other mediators like endotoxin, IL-1, IL-2R, IL-8 might be valuable parameters as well. However there is no possibility to use all these data in clinical practice though they seem to correlate with clinical outcome (Haupt et al. 1996; Reith et al. 1996). Moreover the measurement of endotoxin is difficult and needs a highly experienced laboratory staff and quality control.

2.6
Conclusion

To focus on cytokine measurement alone would be the same as looking to a single liver cell for the function of the liver organ. In conclusion, the "organ-like" immunesystem may be characterised so far by the interaction of markers of the inflammatory potential – like TNF-α or IL-6 – markers for infection and severity of infection – like PCT – and markers for the antiinflammatory response (immunosuppression) as part of the functional status of cells – represented for example as the HLA-DR expression on monocytes.

This is our suggestion for the best parameters presently available. They are valid and sensitive and can be monitored daily in clinical routine.

2.6.1
Options for Treatment of SIRS and Sepsis

The situation in septic patients is complex. Patients may have concomitant diseases and sometimes underwent surgery. These conditions influence the strategy of treatment, that means the use of catecholamines, antibiotics, corticosteroids, organ support therapy (dialysis, hemofiltration a.o.). An additional therapeutic regimen with one drug, such as cytokines and anti-cytokines, leads at best to a moderate improvement of survival rate by modulation of the immune response. The problem is that we do not know at the moment how to best influence this response and what is the exact status of the immune system at the beginning of treatment (Nylen et al. 1992; Marshall 2000).

Another idea was the development of a protective immunisation against bacterial infection. An immunoprophylactic strategy seems to be more promising in clinical practice than treatments that target one mediator of the septic or inflammatory cascade.

This led to the idea of multi-component immunisation strategy in the treatment of infective or septic diseases (Opal et al. 1999).

The application of immunoglobulins (intravenous Immunoglobulins – ivIg) represents such a therapeutic effort to modulate the immune system's response in sepsis. But if we expect that this is the "magic bullet" – as established by Roger Bone, ivIg may not fullfill our hopes (Zanetti and Calandra, 1997). The NIH consensus conference of 1990 did not accept ivIg therapy in sepsis (NIH Concensus conference 1990), however, if we accept the goal "improvement in morbidity" in a complex treatment for the evaluation of a single management, there is a real chance to achieve positive results in sepsis and septic shock. The updated Cochrane meta-analysis (February 2000) of controlled clinical studies stated that there is a benefit for patients treated with polyclonal ivIg's in sepsis and septic shock (Alejandria et al. 2000).

Werdan (1999) described the positive effects of immunoglobulins and the possible mechanism in the treatment of sepsis (Table 2) and pointed out that immunoglobulins are "a useful piece in the therapeutic mosaic of sepsis treatment".

Table 2. Possible mechanisms of ivIg treatment in sepsis (adapted from Werdan 1999)

Toxin inactivation (endo- and exotoxin and superantigen)
     neutralisation
     LPS-clearance
     attenuation of bacterial cell adherance, cell invasion and organ invasion

Stimulation of leukocytes and bactericidal activity in serum
     Enhancement of LPS-induced oxidative burst of neutrophils

Interference with cytokine effects
     Modulation of release of cytokines and antagonists
         pro-inflammation ↓
         anti-inflammation ↑

     cytokines in ivIg-preparations, f. e. TGF
     unspecific antibodies against cytokines

Modulation of complement cascade

Synergistic effects with antibiotics

Table 3. Cochrane analysis of polyclonal intravenous immunoglobulines (ivIg), monoclonal antibodies against endotoxin (Mab) or recombinant anti-cytokines in the treatment of sepsis and septic shock (Alejandria et al. 2000)

	Number of patients	RR (relative risk)	95 % confidence-intervals
IvIg	413	0.60	0.47–0.76
Mab	1736	0.98	0.86–1.12
Anti-cytokine	4318	0.93	0.86–1.01

Cochrane Meta-Analysis

The Cochrane Collaboration Group analyzed 23 high quality studies out of a total of 49 studies published between 1966 and 1999. They found out that there is a significant advantage for the treatment with polyclonal intravenous immunoglobulins – in contrast to treatment with monoclonal antibodies and anti-cytokines (Table 3).

Own Experience with IgM-enriched ivIg

From May 1988 until December 1999 35 patients of our ICU with the diagnosis of severe sepsis or septic shock, according to the ACCP/SCCM-criteria, were treated with additional immunoglobulins (Pentaglobin®). Prerequisite for the immunoglobulin therapy was that the diagnosis was determined within the first 24 hours after admission to the ICU or the very first signs of sepsis. The immunoglobulin dosage was 0.4 ml/kg bodyweight per hour, so that the daily amount of immunoglobulin administered varied – depending on the patient's bodyweight – between 300 ml and 400 ml. The therapy was carried out on 3 consecutive days (Treatment-Group, T-group). Parallely 32 patients with the same diagnosis were treated, however not receiving immunoglobulin therapy

(Control-Group, C-group). In these patients the diagnosis "sepsis or septic shock" did not correspond to our diagnosis/time prerequisites for immunoglobulin therapy, for example because severe sepsis of septic shock had already developed on the patient's previous hospital ward. The APACHE-II score in both groups ranged between 8 and 29 (median 17 pts.) in the T-group and between 8 and 34 (median 17 pts.) in the C-group. There were no differences in age and gender allocation in both groups. The therapeutic regimens on the ICU were standardized for first line antibiotics, the use of colloids, catecholamines and fluid resucitation.

Results

The patients' stay on ICU was 11.6 ± 6.8 days in the Treatment-group and 15.6 ± 5.2 days in the Control-group (n.s.). The overall stay in our hospital was 34.6 ± 13.2 days (Treatment-group) and 39.2 ± 14.4 days in the Control-group (n.s.). The patients' outcome was different in both groups. In the treatment

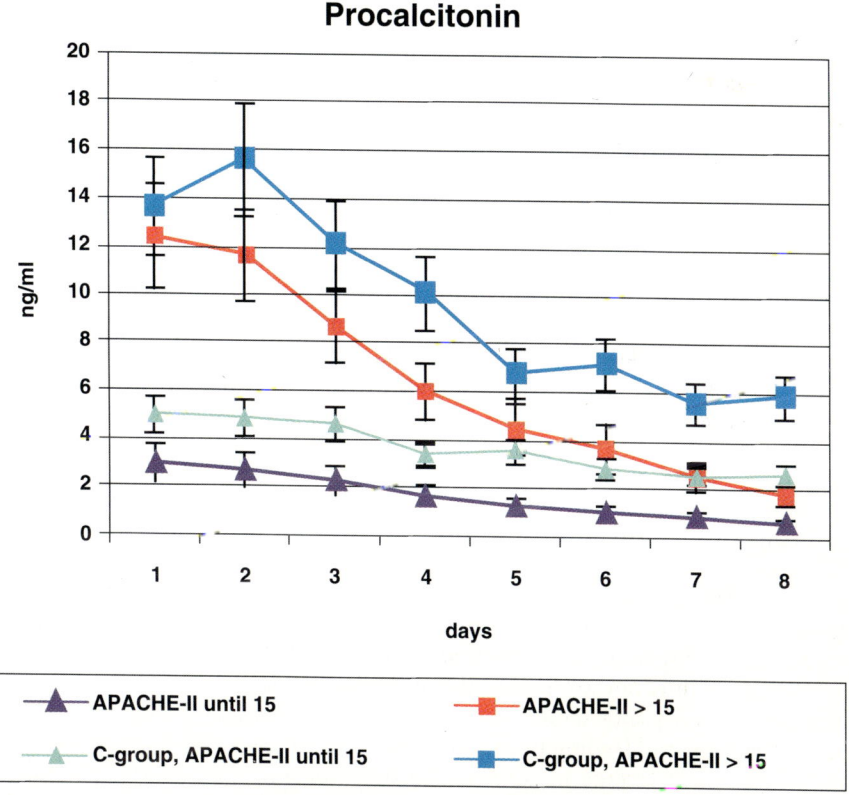

Fig. 5. Procalcitonin follow-up of patients with severe sepsis and septic shock in the therapy and the control group. The data show an early and quick recovery in the treatment group within 4 days on the ICU

group 3 out of 18 patients with severe sepsis died (16.6%) and 4 out of 17 with a septic shock (23.5%). In the control group 5 out of 13 with severe sepsis died (38.5%) and 11 out of 19 with septic shock (57.9%). Summarizing both groups we found a mortality rate of 20% versus 50% (p < 0.05 Chi^2-test). There was a reduction of mortality of 50%.

Looking at relevant laboratory data, there was no difference in leukocytes, SGOT, thrombocytes, albumin, lactate and also the heart rate. But there was an improvement in terms of mean arterial pressure, creatinine and FiO2 in the treatment group. Very interestingly, the follow-up for procalcitonin (Fig. 5) showed a decrease in the treatment group within 4 days.

2.6.2
Future Perspectives

To stratify the risk of patients on an ICU is one of the most important tasks in daily routine. The ACCP/SCCM criteria provide a very easy tool to estimate the patients' condition and a to classify him. Each scoring system gives us the opportunity to reduce complex information from patients to an easy numeric variable, but fails predicting the individual prognosis of a patient. The consensus conference criteria have proved to be a prognostic tool in intensive care medicine. Patients at risk for developing severe sepsis or septic shock encounter the highest mortality rates. For these groups of patients we need more than the standardized regimens of focus sanitation, antibiotics and intensive care mangement. We need an additional fourth column. A number of therapies have been tested for prevention and sepsis control, however only a few approaches demonstrate to be small steps in the difficult way up-hill. Our results with the additional treatment by immunoglobulins are more than satisfactory. The reduction of mortality and the absence of severe adverse events of the drugs are favourable for future concepts. There is no other single crucial measure to influence therapy and outcome in such a positive way. Immunoglobulin treatment has a special impact on: reduction of body temperature (fever, chills), reduction of inflammatory parameters (f. e. procalcitonine), reduction of FiO2 as an indirect sign of better oxygen saturation, stabilisation of mean arterial blood pressure and normalisation of the heart rate (Chen 1996; Grundmann and Hornung 1988; Garbett et al. 1989; Schedel et al. 1991).

The evidence of results like ours is as conclusive as those of small controlled trials (Concato et al. 2000). IvIg may significantly contribute to decrease mortality and morbidity in sepsis patients and therefore plays an important role – now and in future – in an immunmodulatory concert. Many other players in this orchestra may become helpful in various strategies, achieving improvements in organ function and leading to a higher reduction of mortality. Consequently we need more positive data to confirm the statements of meta-analyses in larger trials and with more clinical experience. We are sure that we will not find the "magic bullet" in the future, but the combination of different proven therapies seems to answer to our cry for help in sepsis therapy.

References

Alejandria MM, Lansang MA, Dans LF, Mantaring JBV (1999 and update 2000) Intravenous immunoglobulin for treating sepsis and septic shock (Cochrane-review) The Cochrane Library 3

Assicot M, Gendrel D, Carsin H, Raymond J, Guilbaud J, Bohuon C (1993) High serum procalcitonin concentration in patients with sepsis and infection. Lancet 341: 515

Becker KL, Nash DR, Silva OL, Snider RH, Moore CF (1981) Increased serum and urinary calcitonin levels in patients with pulmonary disease. Chest 79: 211

Beier W (1994) Procalcitonin (ProCt) – ein innovativer Inflammationsparameter mit prognostischen Eigenschaften. Anästh Intensivmed 36: XVIII, (editorial)

Bein T, Unertl K (1993) Möglichkeiten und Grenzen von Score-Systemen in der Intensivmedizin. Anästhesiol. Intensivmed. Notfallmed. Schmerzther. 28: 476–483

Bone RC (1991) The pathogenesis of sepsis. Ann Intern Med 115: 457

Brunkhorst FM, Forycki ZF, Beier W, Wagner J (1993) Discrimination of infectious and non-infectious etiologies of the adult respiratory distress syndrome (ARDS) with procalcitonin immunoreactivity. Clin Intensive Care 3 (suppl); 12

Chen JY (1996) Intravenous immunoglobulin in the treatment of full term and premature newborns with sepsis. J Formos Med Assoc 24: 733–42

Concato J, Shah N, Horwitz RI (2000) Randomized, controlled trials, observational studies, and the hierarchy of research design. NEJM; 342 (25): 1887–1892

Döcke WD, Randow F, Syrbe U, Krausch D, Asadullah K, Reinke P, Volk HD, Kox W (1997) Monocyte deactivation in septic patients: restoration by IFN-γ treatment. Nature Medicine 3: 678–681

Garbett ND, Munro CS, Cole PJ (1989) Opsonic activity of an new intravenous immunoglobulin preparation: pentaglobin compared with sandoglobulin. Clinical Experimental Immunol, 76: 3–12

Goris RJA, Boekhorst TPA, Nuytinck JKS (1985) Multiple organ failure. Arch Surg 118: 1109

Grundmann R, Hornung M (1988) Immunoglobulintherapie in patients with endotoxinemia and postoperative sepsis – a prospective randomized study. Progress in clinical and biological Research 339–349

Haupt W, Fritsche H, Hohenberger W, Zirngibl H (1996) Selective cytokine release induced by serum and separated plasma from septic patients. Eur J Surg 162: 769

Heney D, Lewis IJ, Evans SW, Banks R, Bailey CC, Whicher JT (1992) Interleukin-6 and its relationship to C-reactive protein and fever in children with febrile neutropenia. J Infect Dis 165: 886

Heuer HO, Darius H, Lohmann HF, Meyer J, Schierenberg M, Treese N (1991) Platelet-activating factor type activity in plasma from patients with septicemia and other diseases. Lipids 26: 1381

Huttemeier PC, Ritter EF, Benveniste H (1993) Calcitonin gene-related peptide mediates hypotension and tachycardia in endotoxin rats. Am J Physiol 265: 4767

Joyce CD, Fiscus RR, Wang X, Dries DJ, Morris RC, Prinz RA (1990) Calcitonin related peptide levels are elevated in patients with sepsis. Surgery 108: 1097

Le Gall JR, Lemeshow S, Saulnier F (1993) A New Simplified Acute Physiology Score (SAPS II) Based on a European/North American Multicenter Study. JAMA 270 2957–2963

Marshall JC (2000) Clinical trials of mediator-directed therapy in sepsis: what have we learned? Intensive Care Med. 26: S75–83

Mimos O, Benoist JF, Edouard AR, Assicot M, Bohoun C, Samii K (1998) Procalcitonin and C-reactive protein during the early posttraumatic systemic inflammatory response syndrome. Intensive Care Med 24: 185–188

NIH Consensus conference (1990) Intravenous immunoglobulins. Prevention and treatment of disease. JAMA 264: 3189–3193

Nylen ES, O'Neill WO, Jordan MH et al. (1992) Serum procalcitonin as an index of inhalation injury in burns. Horm Metab Res 24: 439

Opal SM, Cross AS, Bhattacharjee AK, Visvanathan K, Zabriski JB (1999) Immunoprophylaxis against bacterial sepsis. Sepsis 3: 225–234

Rangel-Frausto MS, Pittet D, Costigan, RN, Hwang T, Davis, CS, Wenzel, RP (1995) The natural history of the systemic inflammatory response syndrome (SIRS) JAMA, 273: 117–123

Reist K, Hilfiker O, Stepniewski MS et al. (1996) Sepsis-Score in der operativen Intensivmedizin. Anästhesiol Intensivmed Notfallmed Schmerzther 31

Reith HB, Dittrich H, Haarmann W, Smektala R, Dohle J, Kozuschek W (1996) Adjuvante Therapie der Peritonitis und ihrer septischer Verlaufsformen mit Taurolidin – eine prospektive randomisierte Untersuchung. Chir Gastroenterologie 12: 358

Reith HB, Mittelkötter U, Wagner R, Thiede A (2000) Procalcitonin (PCT) in patients with abdominal sepsis. Intensive Care Med. 26: S 165–169

Rosman C, Grond J, Buurman WA et al. (1993) Fish oil increases the release of tumor necrosis factor and interleukin-6 and has no effect on the incidence of multiple organ failure in rats with peritonitis. Eur J Surg 159: 563

Schedel I, Dreikhausen U, Nentwig B, Hockenschnieder M, Rauthmann D, Balikcioglu S, Coldewey R, Deicher H (1991) Treatment of gram-negative septic shock with an immunoglobulin preparation: a prospective randomized clinical trial. Clinical Care Med, 10: 1104–1113

Werdan K (1999) Immunoglobulins in sepsis: therapeutic use of immunoglobulins. Sepsis 3: 239–245

Zanetti G, Calandra T (1997) Intravenous immunoglobulins and granulocyte colony-stimulating factor for the management of infection in intensive care units. Curr Opin Crit Care 3: 342–347

CHAPTER 3

Microbiological Findings and Antiinfective Treatment Strategies

M. TRAUTMANN and P. M. LEPPER

3.1
Microbiological Diagnosis of Intraabdominal Infections

3.1.1
Overview of Infections

The spectrum of intraabdominal infections includes *primary* processes originating from diseases of the intestinal tract and *secondary* lesions following trauma, surgical interventions, or spontaneous perforations of intestinal organs. A third category of infections are those that result from hematogenous seeding of microorganisms into abdominal organs which may occur during short-lived or prolonged bacteremia or fungemia of extraintestinal origin.

Primary infections include spontaneous or endogenous peritonitis which occurs most often in adult patients suffering from liver cirrhosis. The pathogenesis of this condition involves spontaneous translocation of enteric bacteria into the abdominal cavity where microorganisms find optimal growth conditions in the presence of ascites fluid. Usually, no macroscopic lesions of the intestinal tract can be identified in these cases. In childhood and adolescence, a peculiar disease entity called *juvenile peritonitis* has been described which is often caused by organisms associated with upper respiratory infections such as group A streptococci or pneumococci. It has been speculated that infection of the peritoneal membrane results from hematogenous dissemination of organisms from the respiratory tract. The decreasing incidence of this syndrome has been explained by early antibiotic treatment of infantile respiratory infections.

Secondary infections of the abdominal cavity may result from perforations of intestinal organs which may occur percutaneously (penetrating trauma) or from the lumen of the intestinal tract, as a consequence of benign processes (e.g., Crohn's disease, diverticulitis) or tumor growth. More rarely, the bowel wall may be penetrated by intraluminal foreign bodies or accidentally during endoscopic interventions. In necrotizing pancreatitis, several hypothetical pathways by which bacteria may enter pancreatic and parapancreatic necrosis have been described. These include transmural migration through the colonic bowel wall or from the duodenum via the main pancreatic duct. Another pathomechanism may involve dissemination of bacteria from the large bowel via the lymphatics into ascites fluid or into the portal venous system with subsequent spread to the pancreas. Among the surgical interventions which may be complicated by subsequent infection, colonic surgery carries the highest risk, but small bowel surgery, surgery of the gall bladder and gastric surgery may occasionally also give rise to infection.

Hematogenous dissemination of bacteria or fungi into the spleen, liver or peritoneal membranes is a well-known phenomenon in patients suffering from infectious endocarditis. Multiple miliary or macroscopic abscesses of intestinal organs, mainly of the liver or spleen, may be found in such cases. Furthermore, tuberculosis of the abdominal cavity is often due to hematogenous seeding (e. g. tuberculosis involving the peritoneal membrane with tuberculous exsudate, disseminated tuberculosis of liver and spleen). By contrast, endoluminal tuberculosis of the intestinal tract has become extremely rare in industrialized countries due to the virtual eradication of Mycobacterium bovis. An overview of the most frequent primary or secondary infections of the abdominal cavity is given in Table 1.

The most severe clinical syndrome which may occur as a consequence of any intraabdominal inflammatory process is generalized secondary peritonitis, with or without subsequent abscess formation. Secondary peritonitis is not only a disease of the abdomen but also causes systemic signs and symptoms of infection. The adult respiratory distress syndrome (ARDS), renal failure, or multiple organ failure (MOF) may be a consequence of severe, life-threatening peritonitis. The latter complications are not directly caused by microorganisms but result from the production of microbial toxins which, in turn, stimulate the release of proinflammatory mediators and effector molecules.

Because the majority of secondary abdominal infections are due to migration, translocation or overt spillage of microorganisms from the luminal flora, the spectrum of bacterial and fungal organisms involved often mirrors the flora of the intestinal tract. All microorganisms that are found in the normal intestinal flora such as gram-negative enteric bacilli, enterococci, gram-positive and gram-negative obligate anaerobes and yeasts may also be detected in secondary abdominal infections. Most often, more than one microorganism is isolated, and polymicrobial infections involving ≥3 organisms are frequently encountered. Depending on transport conditions and microbiological culture techniques, up to 30% of the organisms isolated are obligate anaerobes, most often members of the Bacteroides fragilis group. It must be emphasized, however, that in patients who develop abdominal infection after prolonged hospitalization, the normal bacterial flora of the bowel may have undergone significant changes due to suppression of gastric acid secretion, decreased intestinal motility, exogenous infections and/or previous antibiotic therapy. All of these factors may reduce the normal bacterial flora, including anaerobic organisms, and allow typical hospital pathogens such as Pseudomonas aeruginosa, Stenotrophomonas maltophilia, methicillin-resistant staphylococci or Candida spp. to thrive in a changed intestinal ecosystem. Consequently, such "exogenous" organisms may also be found in a variable percentage of abdominal infections. As an example of the flora isolated in three different types of disease, Table 2 gives the spectrum of microorganisms found in acute septic cholecystitis, acute necrotizing pancreatitis and diffuse secondary peritonitis.

Table 1. Primary and secondary infections of abdominal organs

Organ	Disease
Liver	Haematogenous abscess, chologenic abscess
	Amoebic abscess (often multiple)
Gall bladder, gallways	Acute cholecystitis, cholangitis
	Gall bladder empyema
	Parasitic disease (Ascaris, Fasciola), often complicated by secondary bacterial infection
Spleen	Haematogenous abscess
Pancreas	Primary infectious pancreatitis
	during enteric infection (e.g. Salmonella, Campylobacter, Cryptosporidia and other)
	during systemic infection (e.g. Mumps virus, Coxsackievirus and others)
	Secondary pancreatitis
	acute biliary
	alcoholic
	Infected pancreatic necrosis
	Pancreatic abscess, infected cyst
Peritoneum	Primary peritonitis
	Juvenile (hematogenic)
	In liver cirrhosis (by translocation)
	Secondary peritonitis
	traumatic, due to perforation
	postsurgical
	during acute necrotizing pancreatitis
	due to dissemination of pelvic inflammation (Fitz-Hugh-Curtis syndrome, acute perihepatitis[a])
Intestines	Appendicitis
	with empyema
	with perityphlitic abscess
	Mesenteric abscess (perforation, trauma, Crohn's disease)

[a] The Fitz-Hugh-Curtis syndrome may be caused by Chlamydia trachomatis or Neisseria gonorrhoeae, see text.

It should be noted at this point that microorganisms causing primary infections may be significantly different and may not belong to the intestinal flora. Typical examples are hepatic abscesses due to Entamoeba histolytica, peritonitis due to Salmonella typhi as a complication of typhoid fever, or primary peritonitis due to Aeromonas hydrophila (a microorganism found in surface water). Metastatic infections resulting from bacteremia or fungemia of other origin

Table 2. Types of bacteria found at different sites

Organisms	Type of abdominal infection		
	acute cholecystitis (gall fluid) n (%)	secondary peritonitis n (%)	necrotizing pancreatitis n (%)
Gram-positive cocci			
Enterococci	62 (16.4)	5 (4.4)	8 (17.7)
Streptococcus B	3 (0.8)	12 (10.5)	–
oral streptococci	8 (2.1)	25 (21.9)	1 (1.1)
Gram-negative rods			
E. coli	158 (42)	96 (84.2)	24 (53.3)
Enterobacter spp.	34 (9.0)		16 (35.5)
Proteus spp.	18 (4.8)	74 (65)	5 (11.1)
Salmonella spp.	10 (2.7)	(all non E. coli	–
Acinetobacter spp.	5 (1.3)	gram-negative aerobic organisms)	–
Anaerobes			
Clostridium spp.	24 (6.4)	–	–
Bacteroides spp.	4 (1.1)	63 (55.3)	5 (11.1)
Others[a]	51 (13.1)	72 (63.1)	13 (14.3)
Total no. of patients	377 (100)	114 (100)	45 (100)

Adapted from (Beger et al. 1986; Collins et al. 1998; Csendes et al. 1996).
[a] Includes yeasts, ubiquitous mycobacteria and others. Data for secondary peritonitis are derived from pediatric patients suffering mainly from perforated appendicitis.

may be caused by streptococci, e.g. Streptococcus milleri (oral flora), staphylococci (cutaneous or exogenous source), pneumococci (exogenous source), or Salmonella spp. (exogenous source). Acute pelvic inflammatory disease due to Chlamydia trachomatis or Neisseria gonorrhoeae may spread into the abdominal cavity and cause peritonitis with pronounced perihepatitis ("Fitz-Hugh-Curtis syndrome"). In neutropenic patients, the spectrum of such diseases may include a variety of other pathogens such as opportunistic fungi, weakly pathogenic mycobacteria, or protozoa. The present review will focus on postsurgical infections of immunocompetent patients and does not deal with infections involving immunocompromised hosts.

3.1.2
Collection of Specimens, Transport and Microbiological Techniques

Acute cholecystitis and cholangitis. If gall fluid is obtained by sterile puncture, e.g. during surgery, the fluid can be inoculated directly into adequate broth culture media. Most often, aerobic and anaerobic blood cultures bottles will be available, to which the material should be added to result in a final 1:5 to 1:10

mixture of gall fluid to broth. Ideally, culture bottles should be prewarmed to 37 °C and maintained at this temperature after inoculation. Storage at room temperature may reduce sensitivity and should be avoided. If the gall fluid is obtained through the Papilla vateri by endoscopic techniques, the material will be contaminated by pharyngeal and esophageal flora. Therefore, such material should be sent to the laboratory on a swab with transport medium or as native material in a sterile container. In this case, storage must be at 4 °C to prevent overgrowth of contaminants. In acute septic cholangitis and cholecystitis, at least two sets of blood cultures should be taken from different peripheral sites before initiating antimicrobial treament.

Acute necrotizing pancreatitis. Severe pancreatitis requiring surgical intervention is most often due to alcohol abuse or biliary disease. In alcoholic pancreatitis, 60 % of areas of necrosis are bacteriologically sterile, compared to only about half of the necrotic areas in biliary pancreatitis (Beger et al. 1996)). Material for bacteriological examination may be won by percutaneous puncture or during surgery. Specimens taken from the center of the necrosis should be added to aerobic and anaerobic blood culture bottles as described. Alternatively, especially in the case of particulate material, this may be added to Port-a-Cul[R] vials which contain a redox system comprising cysteine and cystine amino acids. This system will reduce atmospheric oxygen after inoculation and firm closure of the screw cap and thus ensure the survival of anaerobic bacteria during storage and transport. Up to 2 ml of fluid or particulate material can be added to one vial. Tissue biopsies should be inoculated into the medium using sterile tweezers and pushed below the agar surface using a sterile swab (Fig. 1). Only in the case of very short transport times (< 1 hr) material should be sent without additives (fluid) or in a small volume of physiological saline (particles, biopsy specimens) in a sterile container. Also, if immediate gram staining is desired, native material must be sent in addition to specimens inoculated into transport media.

Intraabdominal abscesses. The procedure is the same as for pancreatic necrosis. Often, percutaneous drainage of abscesses will be performed, and purulent material may be obtained directly from the first bulk of fluid collected before a suction bag is connected to the tubings. Fluid from hepatic abscesses may be obtained through needle aspiration. Anaerobic cultures are important because obligate anaerobes are nearly always detectable in abdominal abscesses when careful microbiological techniques are employed. The presence of gas collections on CT scans demonstrates the presence of gas-generating anaerobic bacteria (Fig. 2).

Peritonitis. Peritoneal fluid (5 – 10 ml) can be added to blood culture bottles as described above. In addition, direct gram staining is always desirable in order to guide initial therapy. For this purpose, 5 – 10 ml of fluid (depending of the cloudiness of the material) are centrifuged for 15 min at 4000 g. The sediment is resuspended in a small volume of fluid, spread on glass slides, fixed over the flame of a Bunsen burner, and stained with Gram's stain. Alternatively, but with less sensitivity, 50 μl of fluid are spun down in a Cytospin3® centrifuge onto specific

Fig. 1. Application of Port-a-Cul® medium vials for transport of microbiological specimens. A, plain vial; B, vial containing a tissue specimen optimally submerged under the agar surface; C, vial containing a swab; D, vial with purulent liquid filled on top of the agar layer

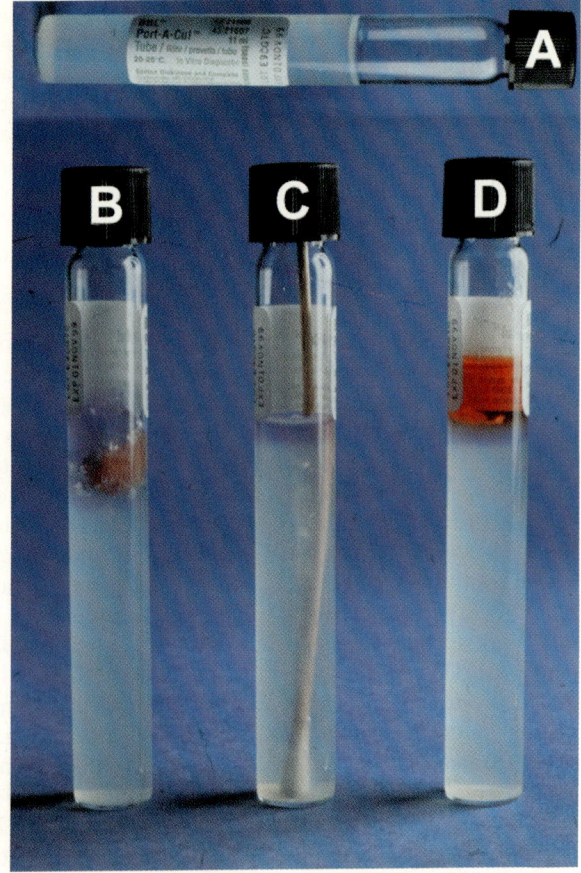

Fig. 2. Abdominal CT scan showing confluent abscesses due to gallbladder perforation in cholecystitis. Gas collections indicate growth of anaerobic organisms (*arrows*)

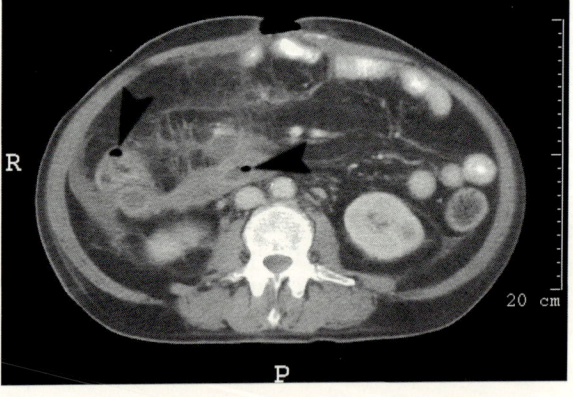

Fig. 3. Patient with continuous abdominal lavage. Fluid collected from tubings should not be added to blood culture bottles but sent to the laboratory in native form

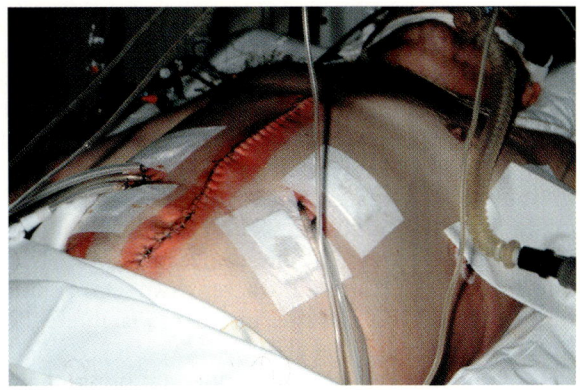

glass slides at 1000 rotations per min for 20 min. In patients treated with continuous peritoneal lavage therapy (Fig. 3), fluid may be collected directly from the lavage tubings. For this purpose, it is important to disinfect the connection piece with a sterile, alcohol-moistened gauze swab, disconnect the tubing, and collect the fluid (~ 10 ml) in a sterile vial which should be kept at 4 °C and sent to the laboratory within 2 hrs. The latter procedure is necessary because the tubing itself may become colonized during lavage therapy, and the spectrum of organisms may include skin contaminants derived from the patient or the nursing staff. Therefore, direct inoculation into blood culture bottles is less advisable. Swabs from the interior of the tubing can be taken if there is a definite suspicion of endoluminal colonization. If the abdominal cavity is opened surgically, i.e. for inspection or débridement, or for targeted insertion of drainage tubings, swabs may be taken directly from sites of inflammation. In this case, Amies or Cary-Blair transport media are suitable for preserving swabs at room temperature for 6 – 12 hrs. Such swabs should not be stored at 4 °C because this will reduce the sensitivity for detection of fastidious bacteria such as streptococci or Neisseria spp.

Suspected septicemia. At least two sets of blood cultures should be taken whenever abdominal infection is associated with signs of systemic infection such as fever, hypotension, or multiple organ dysfunction. It makes no sense to define a specific degree of fever or to wait for chills to occur. Any body temperature ≥ 38 °C is an indication to take blood cultures. Because cultures are often contaminated with skin contaminants, utmost care should be taken to adequately disinfect the skin surface on a 5 × 5 cm area before vein puncture. The skin should be cleansed with gauze swabs moistened with 70 % ethanol or 70 % propanol for at least 1 min. After hygienic hand disinfection with alcohol, gloves should be worn. If non-sterile gloves are used, the site of vein puncture should not be touched after skin disinfection ("non-touch technique"). A total of 10 – 20 ml of blood should be obtained and injected at equal parts into an aerobic and an anaerobic bottle, after careful disinfection of the rubber membrane of the bottles. It is important to change needles before inoculating the bottles because this has been shown to reduce contamination (Spitalnic et al. 1995). Regarding the appropriate number of blood cultures to diagnose septicemia, 88% of cases have been shown to be detected with two separate sets, and 99% of cases with three sets (Washington 1975). However, in a later series, two sets turned out to be sufficient to diagnose 99% of cases (Weinstein et al. 1983). No standard interval between blood cultures can be recommended. Li et al. found that the only significant variable correlating positively with bacteriologic recovery was the volume of blood cultured, whether it be taken at a single or at multiple occasions (Li J et al. 1994). Therefore, if the clinical syndrome is severe enough to warrant an immediate start of antibiotic therapy, two sets of cultures can be taken at the same time, but from different sites in order to facilitate the recognition of contamination by skin flora (Li J et al. 1994).

If blood cultures are taken under antibiotic therapy, it is desirable to collect the blood specimen after the longest possible interval following the last dose of antibiotic. When the patient is clinically stable, an interruption of antimicrobial therapy for 24–48 hrs. is justified. Alternatively, the specimen can be taken directly *before* the next routine i. v. dose of antibiotic. In addition, blood culture media containing antibiotic-neutralizing agents should be preferred. Such media include the Bactec® Plus media containing cationic resins which will bind several classes of antibiotics, or media containing Fuller's earth and charcoal (FAN® medium) which will inactivate antimicrobials by absorption. Although these media enhance the recovery of organisms in antibiotic-treated patients, they do not guarantee complete neutralization of all antimicrobial substances (Weinstein 1996).

It has been debated whether inoculation of an anaerobic bottle is always necessary. However, it has been shown that organisms of the Bacteroides and Clostridium groups are particularly sensitive to oxygen. Among 195 cultures yielding growth of organisms of the Bacteroides group, Cockerill and coworkers found 17 isolates only in the aerobic, 96 only in the anaerobic, and 82 in both bottles (Cockerill et al. 1997). Thus, given the relevance of species of the Bacteroides group for surgical patients, the anaerobic bottle should not be omitted.

Aerobic culture bottles should not be vented by the clinician because this will increase the possibility of contamination. Bottles should arrive in the laboratory within 24 hrs. after inoculation.

Microbiological techniques. In most microbiological laboratories, samples inoculated into blood culture bottles will be processed in automated systems in which bottles are continuously shaken and microbial growth is monitored by detecting CO_2 production by different techniques. Gram staining and appropriate subcultures will be performed immediately after the growth signal has reached a predefined cut-off value. Differentiation of microorganisms is most often possible by biochemical techniques. In rare instances, modern methods such as sequencing of the 16S rRNA region must be used to obtain a definite species diagnosis of fastidious bacteria or rare fungal species (Kolbert and Persing 1999).

From samples arriving in native form, a direct Gram stain may be performed (Fig. 4). Specimens are plated on selective, non-selective and anaerobic agar media.

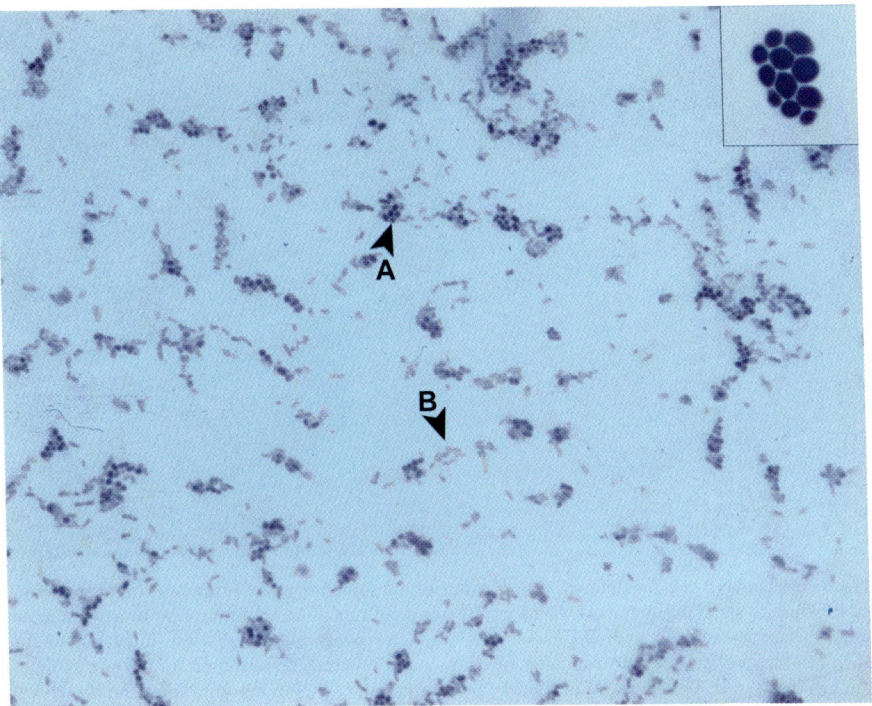

Fig. 4. Gram stain showing the typical mixed flora of secondary peritoneal infection. A, gram-positive cocci, B, gram-negative rods. Insert: Yeast cells

Sensitivity testing of isolates is most often performed by means of the agar diffusion technique. However, in particular in the presence of difficult-to-treat deep-seated infections or septicemia, it is desirable to know the exact minimal inhibitory concentration (MIC) of an antibiotic for relevant pathogens. MIC determination can be performed by broth dilution techniques, but a novel method, the E-test, may be preferable for anaerobic or fastidious organisms and yeasts (Fig. 5). Determination of yeast susceptibility to antifungal drugs by means of the E-test requires some experience, however, good results can be obtained when the media recommended by the American National Committee for Clinical Laboratory Standards (NCCLS) are used (Ruhnke et al. 1996).

3.1.3
Differentiation Between Colonization and Infection

The most difficult question is whether organisms grown on primary cultures are significant for the abdominal process or not. If the material has been won by sterile techniques such as blood cultures, abscess aspiration or puncture of pancreatic necrosis after careful skin disinfection, the organisms recovered may be judged to be causative. Contamination by skin or endogenous flora may occur

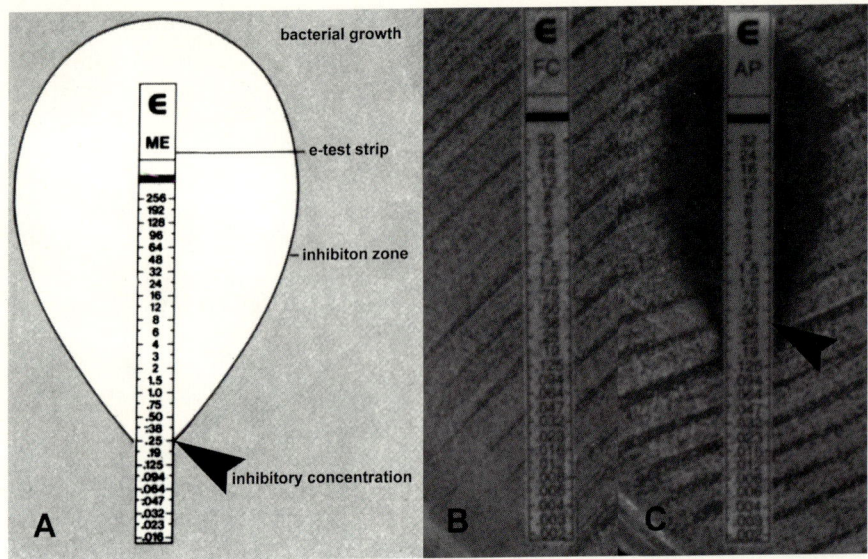

Fig. 5. Erikson (E)-test for determination of antibiotic sensitivity. **A**, demonstration of test principle. A paper strip impregnated with logarithmic dilutions of an antimicrobial is applied to an agar surface inoculated with the test organism. After overnight incubation, diffusion of the antimicrobial substance into the agar medium has occurred, resulting in an elliptic zone of growth inhibition. The minimal inhibitory concentration (MIC) of the antibiotic can be read at the intersection of the ellipse with the paper strip (arrow). **B** and **C**, application of the E-test for sensitivity testing of yeasts. The Candida strain shows resistance to flucytosine (**B**) but sensitivity to amphotericin B (**C**) with a MIC value of 0.38 mg/l (arrow)

when the material is obtained during upper intestinal endoscopy (contamination by oropharyngeal flora), or through percutaneous drainage tubes which may be colonized by skin or hospital flora. Contamination may also occur during open-abdomen treatment of peritonitis or treatment with repeated (e.g. every-day) laparotomies. Table 3 gives an overview of some frequently encountered organisms together with an indication whether they may be regarded as true pathogens or contaminants. If potential contaminants are isolated, the quantity in which they are found may be an indicator of their pathogenic significance.

Regarding blood cultures, it is justified to assume that skin organisms (coagulase-negative staphylococci, propionibacteria, corynebacteria) growing in only one set of two cultures taken separately or in only one bottle represent contamination. In patients with central venous catheters in whom catheter-associated septicemia is suspected or cannot be excluded it is advisable to take two pairs of blood cultures, one through the catheter itself, and one from a peripheral site. When automatic blood culture systems are used which document the time to positivity for every culture, catheter-associated septicemia can be excluded if the peripheral culture becomes positive before or at the same time as the culture taken through the catheter (Blot et al. 1999).

Table 3. Normal habitat of some microorganisms and pathogenetic role in abdominal infection

Organism (species)	Normal habitat	Significance when isolated from abdominal infections
S. aureus	skin, nasal vestibulum	significant
coagulase-negative staphylococci	skin, secondary growth on tubings or intravascular systems	often contaminant
Propionibacterium spp.	skin	often contaminant
Corynebacterium spp.	skin	often contaminant
Viridans streptococci	oral cavity	possibly significant
peptostreptococci	oral cavity	possibly significant
enterococci	large bowel	often significant
Escherichia coli	large bowel	often significant
Other enterobacteriaceae	large bowel	often significant
Salmonella spp.	animal reservoirs, human excretors (S. typhi)	always significant
anaerobic gram-negative rods	large bowel	often significant
Clostridium spp.	large bowel, inanimate environment	often significant
Candida spp.	skin, inanimate environment	often significant
Mycobacterium tuberculosis	other patients	always significant
Opportunistic mycobacteria	inanimate environment	pathogenic in immunosuppressed patients

3.1.4
Interpretation of Sensitivity Tests

The interpretation of antibiotic sensitivity tests requires some knowledge of the pharmacokinetics of drugs and their penetration into abdominal organs. If MIC values can be obtained from the laboratory, these will be helpful to decide whether a given antibiotic or antimycotic drug at the dosage chosen may reach the necessary concentration in blood, organ tissue, abscess fluid, ascitic fluid or peritoneal fluid. Laboratories determining MIC values usually also indicate sensitivity or resistance of the infecting strain by using breakpoints established by the German DIN, the American NCCLS or other committees (Table 4). It must be emphasized that these breakpoints are usually established by judging whether they are exceeded by the mean serum concentration of a drug, while, in general, tissue concentrations are not taken into account. Knowledge of the tissue penetration or gall fluid excretion of a given antibiotic is therefore needed to decide whether a drug is useful for treating infected pancreatic necrosis, peritonitis, abdominal abscesses or cholangitis.

A further important point to note is that staphylococci that are resistant to penicillin G are always also resistant against aminopenicillins, acylureidopeni-cillins and carboxypenicillins. Furthermore, staphylococci resistant to oxacillin are clinically resistant to all other β-lactam antibiotics including carbapenems. These strains, called MRSA (methicillin-resistant S. aureus) or MRSE (methi-cillin-resistant S. epidermidis) are usually sensitive to glycopeptides such as vancomycin and teicoplanin. Some strains may be inhibited by fosfomycin or co-trimoxazole, while aminoglycosides and quinolones are usually not active. Staphylococci that are resistant to glycopeptides have been encountered very rarely, but actually these strains (called GISA, glycopeptide-*intermediately* resistant S. *aureus*) do not represent a problem in Europe.

Enterococci resistant to glycopeptides have spread at the US-American East coast, in particular in New York City. These isolates may also occassionally be encountered in abdominal infections in Europe because they are present in the normal bowel flora of about 1 % of healthy Germans. In patients being treated on

Table 4. Sensitivity breakpoints of commonly used parenteral antibiotics

Drug	Source	MIC (mg/l)		
		sensitive	intermediate	resistant
Amikacin	A	≤ 4	8–16	≥ 32
Ampicillin	A	≤ 2	4–8	≥ 16
Amoxicillin/Clavulanic acid	A	$\leq 2/2$	4/2–8/2	$\geq 16/2$
Cefazolin	A	≤ 4	8	≥ 16
Cefotaxim	A	≤ 2	4–8	≥ 16
Cefoxitin	A	≤ 4	8	≥ 16
Ceftazidim	A	≤ 4	8–16	≥ 32
Ceftriaxon	A	≤ 4	8–16	≥ 32
Cefuroxim	A	≤ 4	8	≥ 16
Ciprofloxacin	A	≤ 1	2	≥ 4
Clindamycin	A	≤ 1	2–4	≥ 8
Fosfomycin	C	≤ 32	–	≥ 64
Gentamicin	A	≤ 1	2–4	≥ 8
Imipenem	A	≤ 2	4	≥ 8
Levofloxacin	B	≤ 2	4	≥ 8
Meropenem	A	≤ 2	4–8	≥ 16
Oxacillin[a]	A	≤ 1	–	≥ 2
Penicillin G[b]	A	≤ 0.125	–	≥ 0.25
Piperacillin	A	≤ 4	8–32	≥ 64
Piperacillin/Tazobactam	A	$\leq 4/4$	8/4–32/4	$\geq 64/4$
Rifampicin	A	≤ 1	2	≥ 4
Tobramycin	A	≤ 1	2–4	≥ 8
Vancomycin	A	≤ 4	8	≥ 16

[a] Oxacillin-resistant staphylococci are judged resistant to all other β-lactams independently of their test results.
[b] Penicillin-resistant staphylococci are judged resistant to all non-inhibitor-protected penicillins.

A: Breakpoint according to German Industrial Standard (DIN, Germany).
B: Breakpoint according to NCCLS, USA.
C: Breakpoint of the Committee of the French Society of Microbiology.

intensive care units, the prevalence of glycopeptide-resistant enterococci may rise to up to 16% (84). In these cases, linezolid or quinupristin/dalfopristin may be the only choice for effective treatment (Chien et al. 2000).

A specific problem is the interpretation of sensitivity tests of yeast isolates such as Candida albicans and other Candida spp. Usually, primary isolates are sensitive to azole antimycotics such as fluconazole, with the exception of some species such as Candida glabrata, Candida krusei and some strains of Candida tropicalis. However, resistance may also develop in Candida albicans during prolonged intravenous therapy in cases of chronic fungal peritonitis or polymicrobial peritonitis with yeasts being part of a mixed flora. Yeast isolates showing fluconazole MIC values of ≤ 8 mg/l are regarded as sensitive to fluconazole, and isolates between 16 and 32 mg/l can still be treated with high doses of 800 mg/day. Strains showing MIC values ≥ 64 mg/l are judged to be clinically resistant. At present, amphotericin B is the only clinical alternative in these cases, pending the introduction of newer, highly active antimycotics such as voriconazole and the echinocandins.

3.2
Empiric Initial Antibiotic Therapy

Before starting antibiotic treatment two questions should be answered: Have all cultures and swabs that can be possibly taken before the start of empiric therapy been obtained, and (Aldridge and Ashcraft 1997) what is the appropriate surgical intervention and is there any need for additional antimicrobial treatment?

In acute cholecystitis, cholangitis, infected pancreatic necrosis, appendicitis and abdominal abscesses, immediate surgical intervention is the treatment of choice. Antibiotics may or may not be given, depending on the clinical situation. For instance, in acute cholecystitis due to gall bladder stones without elevated laboratory parameters indicating biliary obstruction and without visible con crements in the descending gallways, surgery alone is sufficient and antibiotic therapy not needed. If there is evidence of obstruction due to gallway concrements, retrograde endoscopic cholangiography and papillotomy should be performed. In this case, antibiotics should be administered during and after the intervention, because removal of stones from the gallways is only the first step of causative therapy, with cholecystectomy to follow. Similarly, antibiotic therapy may be needed in the presence of a multitude of abdominal abscesses of whom only large ones are drained while smaller ones are left in place and treated conservatively, or before and after surgical treatment of necrotizing pancreatitis.

Acute primary peritonitis in cirrhotic patients may be treated conservatively with antibiotics alone, in conjunction with evacuation of ascitic fluid by single puncture, repeated puncture or continuous drainage. Repeated individual taps may be preferable, because secondary contamination due to drainage tubings is a risk in continuous drainage. In peritonitis during continuous peritoneal dialysis (CAPD) and without significant signs of systemic infection, it may be sufficient to add antibiotics to alternate bags of dialysis fluid. Acute juvenile peritonitis must be treated with systemic antibiotics.

Secondary peritonitis always requires surgical intervention, and antibiotic therapy should be guided by anatomic findings at laparotomy and later modified after the results of microbiological investigations have been obtained. Table 5 summarizes first and second choice options for antibiotic treatment of various abdominal conditions. In some indications, aminoglycosides may be needed which should be applied in the usual single daily dose regimen. The only exception is endocarditis which should be treated with three daily doses.

A variety of randomized, non-randomized comparative or non-comparative studies have been performed using the regimens indicated in Table 5. In primary peritonitis occurring in cirrhotic patients, the third generation cephalosporins such as cefotaxime or ceftriaxone have shown to perform quite well even if treatment periods are limited to 5 days (Javid et al. 1998; Runyon et al. 1991). When comparing the results of two separate studies, amoxicillin/clavulanic acid appears to be less effective than piperacillin/tazobactam, however, due to possible variations in the patient populations studied, differences may have been due to host factors rather than antimicrobial or pharmacodynamic activity (Grange et al. 1990). Nevertheless, piperacillin/tazobactam is microbiologically more active compared to amoxicillin/clavulanic acid and might therefore be preferable, keeping in mind that peritonitis in cirrhotic patients is a condition with high mortality. Given the effective penetration of β-lactams into the peritoneal cavity, the addition of aminoglycosides seems not be necessary. Aztreonam, a drug acting only on gram-negative aerobic organisms, has been shown not to be sufficient as a single-drug treatment in cirrhotic patients because superinfection with gram-positive cocci was noted in a number of cases (Ariza et al. 1986).

In secondary peritonitis, a variety of antibiotic treatment regimens have been studied in conjunction with appropriate surgical interventions. Piperacillin/tazobactam (Ohlin et al. 1999), cefuroxime plus metronidazole (Ohlin et al. 1999), imipenem/cilastatin (Midy et al. 1992), or meropenem (Kanellakopoulou et al. 1993) have been shown to yield comparable results. Some authors felt that initial therapy with a carbapenem might lead to more rapid recovery and somewhat lower total costs although the differences measured were small. The carbapenems have the additional advantage that they do not liberate large amounts of endotoxin during the disintegration of bacteria, a phenomenon that will be discussed later. Therefore, the initial use of imipenem/cilastatin or meropenem may be justified in individual patients. However, in specialized intensive care units caring for many patients with secondary peritonitis, the wide-spread use of imipenem as a first-line agent will lead to rapid emergence of resistant gram-negative bacteria, and to selection of Stenotrophomonas maltophilia. Piperacillin/tazobactam or a cephalosporin combined with metronidazole should be the first choices in this setting. Similar considerations hold true for treatment of abdominal abscesses.

Table 5. Options for empiric initial antibiotic therapy of intraabdominal infections

Disease	microbial etiology	Empirical antibiotic therapy	
		first choice	alternative
Acute cholecystitis, acute cholangitis	enterobacteriaceae, enterococci, anaerobes (Bacteroides spp., Clostridium spp.)	Acylureidopenicillin plus metronidazole, or piperacillin/ tazobactam	cephalosporin 3a plus metronidazole
Necrotizing pancreatitis with infected necrosis, abscess	enterobacteriaceae, enterococci, S. aureus, S. epidermidis, anaerobes, Candida spp.	piperacillin/ tazobactam, or carbapenem, or quinolone 2 plus metronidazole	cefoxitin
Acute appendicitis	enterobacteriaceae, enterococci, anaerobes	preoperative prophylaxis only (cephalosporin 2; 1 dose)	amoxicillin/ clavulanic acid (1 dose)
Primary peritonitis in pts. with liver cirrhosis	enterobacteriaceae, Aeromonas hydrophila, streptococci, enterococci, rarely anaerobes (<2%)	cephalosporin 3a	piperacillin/ tazobactam
Juvenile primary peritonitis	α-hemolytic streptococci, pneumococci, staphylococci, enterobacteriaceae	cephalosporin 3a	amoxicillin/ clavulanic acid
Secondary peritonitis	enterobacteriaceae, Bacteroides spp., P. aeruginosa, yeasts	piperacillin/ tazobactam plus aminoglycoside, or cephalosporin 3b plus metronidazole	carbapenem, or ciprofloxacin plus metronidazole, or cefoxitin plus aminoglycoside
Peritonitis during CAPD	staphylococci, enterobacteriaceae, P. aeruginosa, rarely yeasts	vancomycin plus aminoglycoside (intraperitoneally)	cefazolin plus aminoglycoside (intraperitoneally)
Fitz-Hugh-Curtis syndrome	Chlamydia trachomatis or Neisseria gonorrhoeae	quinolone 2	macrolide plus cephalosporin 3, tetracycline plus cephalosporin 3
Abdominal abscess	enterobacteriaceae, enterococci, streptococci, Bacteroides spp.	piperacillin/ tazobactam ± aminoglycoside, or cephalosporin 3a plus metronidazole	carbapenem, or cefoxitin plus aminogylcoside

Notes: Cephalosporin 2, second generation cephalosporin (e.g. cefuroxime, cefotiam); cephalosporin 3a, third generation cephalosporin without antipseudomonal activity (e.g. cefo-taxime, ceftriaxone); quinolone 2, second generation quinolone (e.g. ciprofloxacin, ofloxacin). Note: levofloxacin, a third generation quinolone, may be preferable to ofloxacin.

3.3
Organism-Targeted Specific Antimicrobial Therapy

After the results of cultures have been obtained, treatment should be modified to include all pathogens judged to be significant. Usually, the sensitivity data provided by the laboratory will help the clinician to decide which drugs to use. However, some important points should be noted in order to avoid mistakes commonly being made during routine intensive care therapy.

One important point is that antibiotics whose antimicrobial spectrum covers obligate anaerobes should not be combined with metronidazole. The latter drug is a potent antianaerobic substance with particularly high activity against Bacteroides and Clostridium spp. However, it has some immunosuppressive activity on T lymphocytes and should be avoided when possible. Metronidazole may be given in combination with second and third generation cephalosporins, second and third generation quinolones and with amino- or acylureidopenicillins because these drugs lack activity against gram-negative anaerobic rods of the Bacteroides family. However, treatment periods with metronidazole should be limited to approximately 7 days. When amino- or acylureidopenicillins are combined with a β-lactamase inhibitor such as clavulanic acid or tazobactam, addition of metronidazole is not necessary because such inhibitor combinations confer excellent activity against β-lactamase-producing anaerobic rods.

Another point is the combination of two β-lactam agents. Although such regimens have been studied and advocated in the 70s and early 80s it has now become apparent that some first generation cephalosporins, aminopenicillins, as well as cefoxitin and imipenem may act as strong inducers of β-lactamases of many gram-negative bacterial species including enterobacteriaceae and Pseudomonas aeruginosa (Bongaerts et al. 1998). Acylureidopenicillins are known to act as weak inducers. Therefore, combinations including a cephalosporin and a broad-spectrum penicillin, or combinations between a cephalosporin and a carbapenem should be avoided. Clinical failures due to induction of β-lactamases by such combinations have been described (Livermore 1987). Useful, potentially synergistic combinations are those between β-lactams and carbapenems on one hand, and aminoglycosides on the other hand. Combinations between β-lactams and quinolones may act in an additive manner and can be recommended if nephrotoxicity due to aminoglycosides is a problem.

A final point is that infections due to Pseudomonas aeruginosa should always be treated with two active antibiotics which are potentially synergistic or at least additive. Such combinations include piperacillin/tazobactam plus an antipseudomonal aminogylcoside such as tobramycin or amikacin, or an antipseudomonal cephalosporin such as ceftazidime with one of these aminogylcosides. Also, ciprofloxacin can be used as a combination partner, but other quinolones should be avoided because their antipseudomonal activity is weaker compared to that of ciprofloxacin. This is also true for upcoming drugs such as moxifloxacin, gemifloxacin and gatifloxacin.

For specific treatment of yeast infections or polymicrobial infections with participation of yeasts, fluconazole is used as the drug of first choice. The usual dose in patients without impairment of renal or hepatic function is 800 mg which may be given in a single daily dose, or twice daily. In patients with hepatic cirrhosis, the dose may be the same for Child A and B stages, i.e. those patients without additional impairment of renal function (Ruhnke et al. 1995). Apart from Candida albicans, treatment with such doses will also reach ~ 70% of the strains of Candida glabrata and Candida tropicalis which are less sensitive to fluconazole. Candida krusei is usually not sensitive. Amphotericin B is the drug of choice for infections due to fluconazole-resistant yeasts. Other families of fungi are rarely involved in abdominal infections. The duration of treatment of fungal infections is a matter of debate; we prefer treatment periods of 12–14 days after which new cultures will be obtained.

The dosage of antimicrobial agents in renal insufficiency and during hemo-dialysis and hemofiltration is a topic that goes beyond the scope of this chapter. Because most intensive care clinicians prefer treatment with continuous renal replacement therapy, the reader is referred to the review by Reetze-Bonorden et al. (Reetze-Bonorden et al. 1993).

3.4
Limits and Problems of Antibiotic Therapy

3.4.1
Tissue Penetration of Drugs

As mentioned above, usually much information is available regarding the serum pharmacokinetics of drugs while little data exist about bile excretion, penetra-tion into abscesses, or penetration into infected and/or necrotic pancreatic tissue. Some information may be gathered from animal experimental studies which have been performed with models of necrotizing pancreatitis or intra-abdominal abscesses. The following paragraphs will summarize some of these data. It should be kept in mind, however, that, in the clinical situation, patholo-gic conditions such as bile obstruction or massive hyperemia due to inflamma-tion may alter the pharmacokinetic behaviour of drugs.

Bile excretion is regarded to be important for antibiotics used to treat infec-tions of the gall bladder and biliary tree. A common way to express the amount of substance excreted in the bile is the ratio between peak drug levels that have been measured in human bile and peak serum levels. In Table 6, these ratios are summarized for antibiotics commonly used in bilary surgery. It can be seen that some drugs such as mezlocillin, piperacillin with or without tazobactam, ciprofloxacin and ceftriaxone are very effectively excreted through the bile. However, as can be seen in the case of ceftriaxone, biliary fluid levels will be significantly lower in cases of obstructive jaundice. Although this has not been examined in detail for other antibiotics, excretion may be similarly reduced, a phenomenon which should be kept in mind when treating biliary infection in the presence of obstruction. Due to its high biliary excretion, ceftriaxone has been associated with formation of sludge in the gall bladder, however, in most cases this finding has not been clinically significant.

Table 6. Bile excretion of selected antibiotics

Drug	Dose (i.v.)	peak serum level (mg/l)	% biliary excretion[a]
Ampicillin/sulbactam	2 g/1 g	35/16	> 100
Mezlocillin	4 g	80	1000–6000
Piperacillin	4 g	320	100–6000
Piperacillin/tazobactam	4 g/0.5 g	320/28	> 100
Cefazolin	1 g	188	29–300
Cefuroxim	1.5 g	100	35–80
Cefoxitin	1 g	110	280
Cefotaxime	2 g	200	15–75
Ceftazidime	2 g	120	13–54
Ceftriaxon	2 g	220	200–500 (normal bile flow) 40 (bile obstruction)
Imipenem	1 g	60	minimal
Meropenem	1 g	49	3–300
Amikacin	7.5 mg/kg	38	30
Gentamicin	1.25 mg/kg	4-8	10–60
Tobramycin	1.25 mg/kg	4-8	10–60
Ciprofloxacin	400 mg	4.6	2800–4500
Ofloxacin	400 mg	5.2–7.2	210–1886
Levofloxacin	500 mg	6.2	see ofloxacin
Metronidazole	500 mg	20–25	100
Rifampin	600 mg	7.0	10,000
Co-trimoxazole	1600 TMP/800 mg SMX	TMP 9; SMX 105	40–70
Vancomycin	1 g	20–50	50
Teicoplanin	6 mg/kg	112	minimal

Table after (Gilbert et al. 1999), with modifications. [a] Percentage value calculated as follows: Peak levels measured in bile, divided by peak serum level, × 100.

Penetration of drugs into pancreatic necrosis has been examined in human samples and in animal models. In a study with patients who underwent needle aspirations or surgery of pancreatic necrosis at predefined intervals after antibiotic infusion, it could be shown that aminoglycosides penetrated poorly into necrotic tissue while pefloxacin and metronidazole penetrated very efficiently. Mezlocillin and imipenem/cilastatin penetrated to a variable extent and did not always reach the MIC values of commonly encountered microorganisms (Bassi et al. 1994). In spite of the excellent penetration of pefloxacin, however, it appeared inferior to imipenem/cilastatin in a later clinical trial performed by the same group of authors (Bassi et al 1998). In a study with 89 patients undergoing pancreatic surgery, Buchler et al. found relevant drug concentrations 120 min after administration for mezlocillin, piperacillin, imipenem and metronidazole. These authors divided antibiotics into three groups with respect to their ability to penetrate into pancreatic tissue: Group A, substances with low tissue concentration (the aminoglycosides), group B, drugs with tissue concentrations sufficient to inhibit some but not all bacteria in pancreatic infection (mezlocillin, piperacillin, ceftizoxime, cefotaxime), and group C, antibiotics with high pancreatic tissue levels and high bactericidal activity against organisms commonly isolated in necrotizing pancreatitis (ciprofloxacin, ofloxacin, and imipenem) (Buchler et al. 1992). The efficient penetration of ciprofloxacin into pancreatic tissue and juice was later confirmed by Isenmann et al. (Isenmann et al 1994). Therefore, although imipenem and ciprofloxacin are costly antibiotics, the use of these agents in necrotizing pancreatitis seems to be indicated.

For abdominal abscesses, antibiotic penetration into pus has been examined in animal experimental studies while concentrations in humans are not available. Individual cases or small series in which a complete resolution of minor abscesses was achieved with antibiotics alone have been published (Gorenstein et al. 1994). Larger abscesses are generally drained by percutaneous puncture, most often under ultrasonic or CT guidance. In addition, antibiotics are given to prevent the effects of spilling of microorganisms into the abdominal cavity. For this purpose, piperacillin/tazobactam, mezlocillin plus sulbactam, ampicillin plus sulbactam, or clindamycin plus aztreonam appear to be clinically equivalent. It should be noted that aminoglycosides not only penetrate poorly into abscesses but also loose much of their antibacterial activity due to the acid pH and low oxygen tension in the abscess environment. Therefore, other antibiotics with activity against aerobic gram-negative organisms such as the quinolones should be used as a combination partner for β-lactam/inhibitor combinations if judged to be necessary. In particular, it has been shown for ciprofloxacin that this agent retaines its antibacterial activity in the acid and anaerobic environment of purulent abscess fluid (Bryant and Mazza 1989). Once novel fourth generation quinolones such as moxifloxacin have been marketed, these agents may be useful for monotherapy of abdominal infections because their spectrum includes both gram-positive cocci, gram-negative aerobic rods, and anaerobic bacteria. For instance, moxifloxacin has been shown to exhibit activity against 91% and 96% of 410 clinically relevant anaerobic isolates at concentrations of 2 and 4 mg/l, respectively (Aldridge 1997).

In secondary bacterial peritonitis, cephalosporins such as cefotaxime penetrate very effectively into peritoneal exsudate reaching levels corresponding to those in the serum a few hours after i.v. infusion (Runyon et al. 1991). Similar data have been generated for ciprofloxacin (Hoogkamp-Korstanje 1995), while earlier studies with mezlocillin indicated impaired penetration with coverage of only about 75% of organisms isolated during postsurgical peritonitis (Wittmann et al. 1982). The activity of imipenem seems to be somewhat impaired in purulent peritoneal exsudate (Konig et al. 1998). Newer acylureidopenicillins in combination with β-lactamase inhibitors or quinolones should therefore be preferred. For fungal peritonitis, fluconazole remains the drug of choice because its penetration ratio through the peritoneal barrier is nearly 100%. However, this should be also taken into consideration when peritonitis is treated by continuous lavage therapy which will remove large amounts of systemically administered fluconazole from the circulation. In such cases, it is advisable to add 30–40 mg/l of fluconazole to each volume of lavage fluid in order to stabilize serum concentrations at this level. Amphotericin B penetrates very poorly into the abdominal cavity and should not be used to treat fungal peritonitis, unless resistance against azole drugs has emerged.

Although these data indicate that effective therapy of intraabdominal infections should be possible it must be taken into consideration that pharmacokinetic factors may change in the course of any severe abdominal disease. For gall bladder and biliary diseases, motility of the gall bladder and unimpaired flow of gall fluid are a prerequisite for antibiotic excretion through the descending gall ways. This will often not be the case in chronic cholecystitis with bladder wall thickening or in the presence of duct stones. Therefore, cholecystectomy and complete restoration of bile flow by endoscopic or surgical techniques are the primary measures to be taken in these cases. In peritonitis, the peritoneal membrane will undergo thickening and may be covered with large amounts of fibrin during prolonged open-abdomen or lavage treatment, thus impairing peritoneal and mesenteric circulation and antibiotic distribution. Finally, although the data by Buchler et al. indicate effective penetration of drugs into pancreatic tissue this may not be the case in the center of large necrotic areas not accessible to any blood flow (Buchler et al. 1992). Therefore, if failures of antibiotic therapy occur, the above-mentioned anatomical and pathophysiological factors should be considered.

3.4.2
Development of Resistance

This will not be a problem during short-term treatment of cholecystitis, cholangitis or abdominal abscesses. However, during prolonged therapy of chronic secondary peritonitis, resistance may be induced by certain classes of β-lactams, mainly in enteric gram-negative bacteria. Thus, β-lactamase-producing Klebsiella or Enterobacter spp. may be selected. A common phenomenon is the emergence of Pseudomonas aeruginosa and/or Stenotrophomonas maltophilia as secondary colonizers during prolonged treatment. Data generated by hospital epidemiologists have shown that these bacteria thrive in the hospital water systems and most likely gain access to the patient through procedures such as oral hygiene, wound care or body washing. For instance, tap water harbouring Stenotrophomonas maltophilia may be used to wash the abdominal skin, and the organism may reach abdominal lavage tubings by spillage of water.

Generation of resistance to fluconazole usually needs prolonged exposure to the drug for months to years. Most of these cases have therefore been described in HIV-infected patients. However, recently, we observed a case of secondary peritonitis due to Candida utilis after perforation of a duodenal ulcer (Trautmann et al., unpublished observation). In this case, resistance to fluconazole developed after an ineffective 4-week treatment period. It should be noted, however, that the pharmacokinetic of fluconazole was poorly predictable in this patient who underwent continuous hemodialysis with hemofiltration (CVVHDF) in addition to peritoneal lavage therapy. Therefore, therapeutic drug levels in the peritoneal exsudate may not have been obtained.

3.4.3
Endotoxin Release by Antibiotics

A significant percentage of cases of secondary peritonitis are complicated by signs of systemic inflammation. In some instances, patients proceed to develop hypotension, shock, the adult respiratory distress syndrome, and multiorgan failure. It is widely accepted that the liberation of bacterial endotoxin (lipopolysaccharide, LPS) is a major component of the pathophysiological cascade leading to tissue and organ injury.

Although the effects of bacterial endotoxin have been known for decades, it has become apparent only recently that antibiotics may play a role in its liberation from the cell wall of gram-negative bacteria. Endotoxin may be liberated spontaneously during multiplication of microorganisms, however, its release has been shown to be precipitated by the antibiotic-induced destruction of bacteria. Compared to bacterial cell-bound endotoxin, soluble endotoxin released from bacteria by the action of antibiotics may have an up to 50fold increased biological activity. Clinically, this phenomenon was first noted during treatment of typhoid fever in the 1940s, when some patients showed rapid deterioration of their clinical condition after antibiotic administration. The pathophysiological basis of this phenomenon was not understood because assay systems to detect or measure endotoxin in plasma or body fluids were not available. After the development of the Limulus amoebocyte lysate (LAL) assay in the late 1960s, Levin and others were able to show that free endotoxin could be detected in the systemic circulation in such cases (Levin et al. 1970). In the 80s, Shenep et al. were the first to show that antibiotics that act on the cell wall of gram-negative organisms liberated greater amounts of endotoxin compared to drugs acting on protein synthesis such as the aminoglycosides (Shenep et al. 1985).

During the last decade, it became clear that various classes of cell-wall active drugs also exhibit differences in their endotoxing-liberating potential. The degree of endotoxin liberation caused by β-lactam antibiotics appears to be best predicted by their influence on bacterial morphology. Third generation cephalosporins and monobactams such as aztreonam are known to induce the formation of filamentous bacterial cell forms which have a high biomass and thus liberate large amounts of endotoxin when finally being lysed. Conversely, drugs that are quickly bactericidal or induce the development of roundish bacterial cells – called spheroplasts – may be associated with low endotoxin release. Spheroplast formation is triggered mainly by carbapenem antibiotics and appears to be related to the preferential binding of this class of agents to penicillin-binding protein 2 (PBP2) of gram-negative bacteria. The formation of filaments, as seen e.g. in the presence of third generation cephalosporins, appears to be caused by their preferential binding to PBP3. The morphology of spheroplasts and filaments is shown in Fig. 6.

Fig. 6. A, electron micro-
scopic morphology of
untreated E. coli cells;
B, cells treated with ceftazidime (filamentous form)
and C, cells treated with
imipenem (spheroplasts)

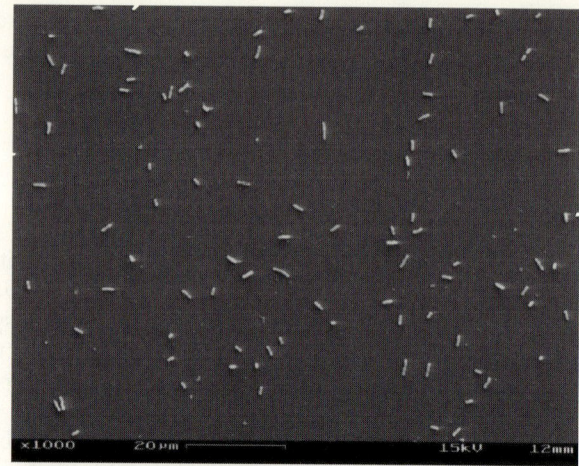

A

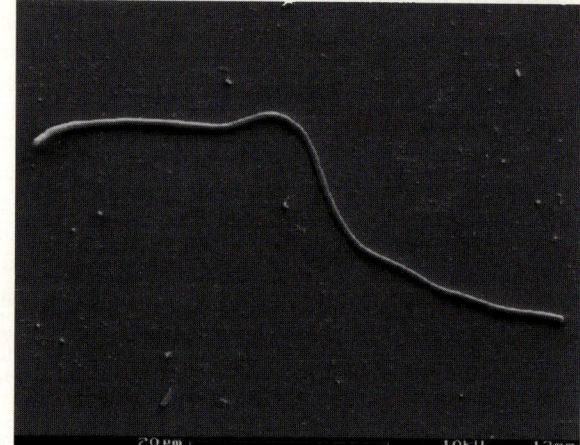

B

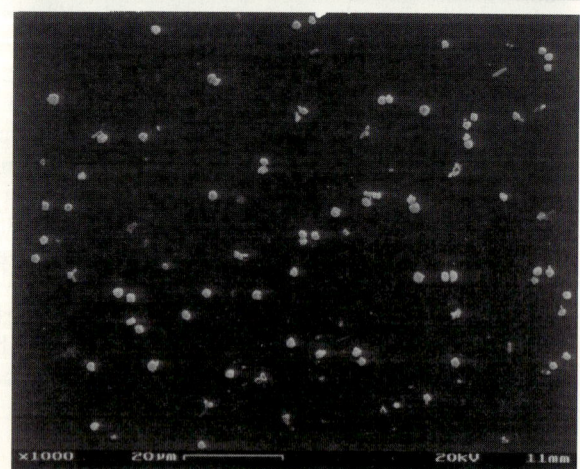

C

It has been debated whether the differential release of endotoxin due to various classes of β-lactam (and other) agents correlates with pathophysiological events. Recently, we were able to show in an in vitro system that this was in fact the case (Trautmann et al. 1999). When E. coli bacteria were treated with three different concentrations of ceftazidime (representing a PBP3-specific antibiotic), imipenem (representing a PBP2-specific antibiotic) and ciprofloxacin (not binding to PBPs), we observed a considerable release of endotoxin in the culture treated with ceftazidime in contrast to those treated with imipenem and ciprofloxacin, when rapidly bactericidal concentrations such as 10 × the MIC were used (Fig. 7, panel A). When the supernatants of these cultures (containing the soluble endotoxin) were removed and pipetted onto human monocytes, these cells were stimulated to release proinflammatory mediators such as TNFα (Trautmann et al. 1999). From Fig. 7, panel B it is evident that the cultures containing much endotoxin also released the highest amounts of TNFα, which proves that the endotoxin was functionally active.

There have been two randomized trials of antibiotic-induced endotoxin release with patients suffering from well defined diseases due to gram-negative

Fig. 7. Correlation between antibiotic-induced endotoxin release and biological activity. A, amounts of free endotoxin released in vitro from E. coli cells after 4 h exposure to ciprofloxacin, imipenem and ceftazidime. Endotoxin (LPS) concentrations were determined by Limulus assay in the supernatants of E. coli cultures exposed to the indicated concentrations of antibiotics (MIC, minimal inhibitory concentration). B, TNFα release from human monocytes exposed to the culture supernatants shown in panel A. TNFα levels correspond to LPS concentrations (coefficient of correlation 0.94), proving the functional activity of antibiotic-liberated LPS. After (Trautmann et al. 1999)

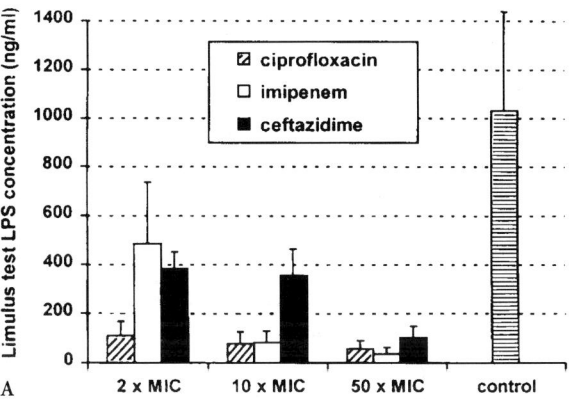

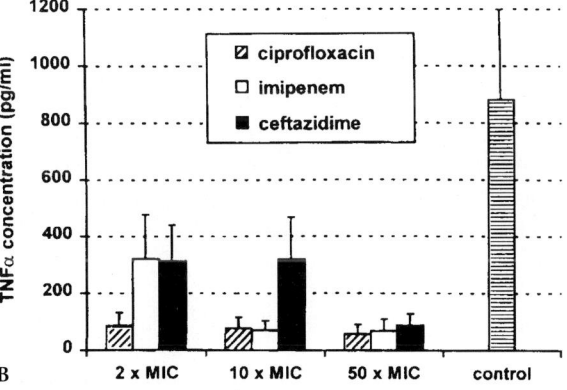

organisms in which the groups were sufficiently homogeneous to allow statistical conclusions. In one study, patients with urosepsis were treated, and a clinical advantage of imipenem therapy was noted which caused a more rapid defervescence compared to ceftazidime, correlating with reduced endotoxin liberation (Prins et al. 1995). More recently, Simpson et al. studied patients suffering from melioidosis, a disease caused by the gram-negative rod-shaped organism Burkholderia pseudomallei, occurring on the Malaysian peninsula. In the latter trial, 68 patients were randomized to receive imipenem or ceftazidime, and the imipenem-treated patients showed lower systemic endotoxin levels after the first administration of antibiotic. The overall survival rate, however, was virtually the same in both groups (Simpson et al. 2000).

Although these studies seem to indicate that the role of specific antibiotics for endotoxin release in patients is negligible, there have been strong hints from an earlier study by Mock et al. that the selection of antibiotics plays a role for clinical outcome in septic surgical patients (Mock et al. 1995). In 334 severely injured trauma patients, 80% of whom developed some manifestation of gram-negative infection, the authors examined the effect of PBP3-specific versus non-PBP3-specific antibiotics on overall in-hospital mortality. In 78 patients receiving PBP3-specific antibiotics (aztreonam, cefotaxime, or ceftazidime), mortality was 17% as compared to a mortality of 8% in the group of 256 patients receiving other antimicrobials (p = 0.02). This difference became even more pronounced when only those subgroups of patients were evaluated in which the antibiotics were active against infection-associated pathogens (Table 7). A drawback of this analysis was the fact that, although the initial study (designed to test the effect of interferon-γ in trauma patients) was prospective, the analysis of the effects of antibiotic treatment was done by retrospective examination of patient charts (Mock et al. 1995). Nevertheless, together with the in vitro data these findings indicate that endotoxin liberation by certain classes of antibiotics in severely compromised patients should not be neglected. Further studies are clearly needed to elucidate this phenomenon.

Various authors have shown that endotoxin is present both in plasma and peritoneal exsudate during severe peritonitis. Due to technical limitations of endotoxin determination it has never become clear to what extent elevated endotoxin levels predict a detrimental clinical outcome or death (Fugger et al. 1990). Nevertheless, some clinicians have propagated the use of an endotoxin-

Table 7. Influence of antibiotic class on mortality in septic trauma patients

Patient group	Mortality (%)
Total PBP3-group (ceftazidime, cefotaxime, aztreonam)	13/78 (18.7)
Subgroup with negative blood culture	10/66 (15.2)
Non PBP3-group (e.g. aminopenicillins, aminoglycosides, imipenem and others)	20/256 (7.8)
Subgroup with negative blood culture	12/234 (5.1)

After (Mock et al. 1995).

binding agent, taurolin, as an addition to lavage fluids in the surgical treatment of peritonitis. Taurolin is a disinfectant substance comprising a thiadiazine structure and exhibits both bactericidal and endotoxin-binding activities in the peritoneal cavity, when added at concentrations of 0.5–2% to lavage fluid. The substance appears to have no detrimental effects on influx and function of phagocytic cells (Billing et al. 1992). However, in a recently performed rat study of artificially induced fecal peritonitis, taurolin reduced plasma and peritoneal exsudate endotoxin levels, but did not exhibit bactericidal activity nor lower mortality. By contrast, addition of imipenem/cilastatin to the lavage fluid reduced not only endotoxin levels, but also bacterial growth, abscess formation and mortality (Rosman et al. 1999). Therefore, taurolin may be unnecessary if imipenem/cilastatin is used for treatment of peritonitis. It was not examined in this study whether systemic treatment with imipenem/cilastatin might have the same effect.

Taken together, it can be said that endotoxin is regularly present both in the plasma and peritoneal exsudate of patients suffering from severe secondary peritonitis. The technical difficulties associated with endotoxin determination and the fluctuation of endotoxin levels in plasma have so far prevented the use of the LAL assay to predict the outcome of patients or to guide treatment. Knowing the pathophysiological effects of endotoxin, however, it appears reasonable to assume that all interventions suitable to reduce the endotoxin burden in the peritoneal cavity may be beneficial for the patient. Choosing antibiotics that are known to liberate only minor amounts of endotoxin while effecting bacterial killing may be beneficial although randomized prospective clinical trials in surgical patients have yet to be performed. An important point is that antibiotic therapy should be clearly stratified (according to PBP3-specific and non PBP3-specific agents) in all trials designed to study the influence of anti-endotoxin agents such as monoclonal antibodies or immunoglobulins. Pending the results of such studies, surgical interventions suitable to reduce endotoxin generation in the peritoneal cavity should include lavage therapy, use of systemic antimicrobials to prevent further bacterial growth, and possibly the use of taurolin to bind existing endotoxin.

3.5
Options for Improved Antiinfective Treatment Strategies

3.5.1
Overview of Immunotherapeutic Approaches

Surgical interventions and antimicrobial chemotherapy reach their limit when the patient with complicated intraabdominal infection proceeds to develop volume-refractory hypotension, the adult respiratory distress syndrome, renal failure, and finally multiorgan failure. It is this scenario known to every intensive care physician that has acted as a constant stimulus to look for additive or alternative treatment modalities.

Once the pathophysiological relevance of endotoxin had been accepted, attempts were made to neutralize endotoxin in the circulation by infusing

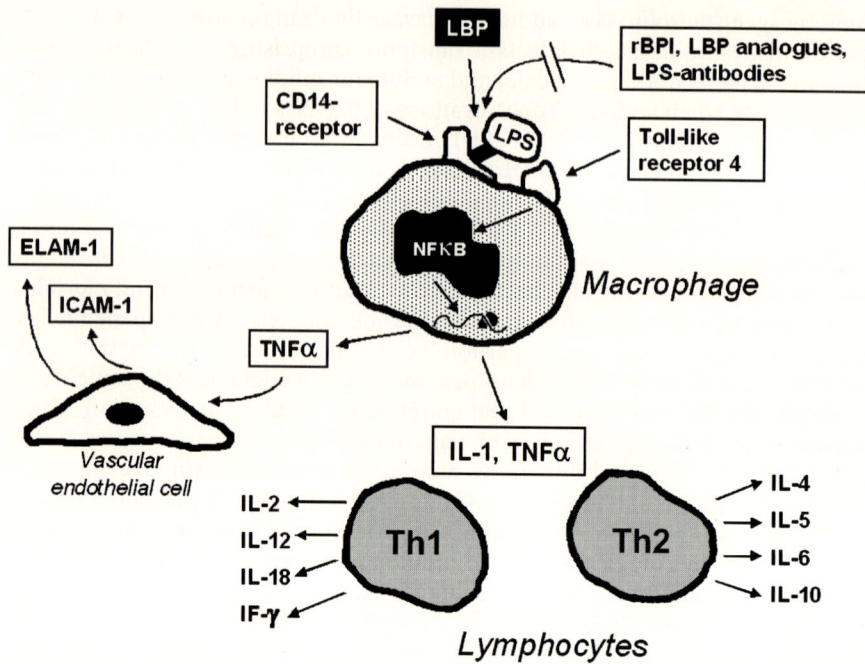

Fig. 8. Scheme of LPS interaction with the human macrophage. LPS binding to the cell surface occurs via the CD14 receptor, with LBP acting as a bridging molecule. Immunoglobulins, LBP analogues, or recombinant BPI can prevent LPS binding to CD14. The initiation of the intracellular signalling cascade occurs through the Toll 4 receptor

specific or polyclonal antibodies, or by abrogating the secondary effects of endotoxin action. Since it was known that the endotoxin action started by binding of the molecule to the CD14 receptor of monocytes, some authors focussed on inhibiting this binding process by adding recombinant soluble CD14 or by diverting LPS from the receptor by means of the bactericidal permeability increasing protein (BPI) which has become available commercially as a recombinant product. These options appear quite promising and will be discussed in detail at the end of this chapter. Other investigators focussed on proinflammatory cytokines such as TNFα and IL-1 that are liberated after processing of LPS by the macrophage. An overview of the sites of LPS binding, the molecules involved and their target cells is given in Fig. 8.

Although there is an excessive number of experimental and clinical studies that have been dealing with the counteraction of proinflammatory mediators released by target cells of endotoxin, the disappointing denominator of all of them is that, beyond appropriate antibiotics, a single immunotherapeutic agent is not able to reduce mortality in severe sepsis and septic shock. Table 8 summarizes studies that had been performed until 1998. It becomes clear that mortality has actually remained at a level of about 35–50%, which is the same as it has been in the 1960s.

Table 8. Mortality in sepsis trials

Type of trial	No. of trials	Total no. of patients	Mortality	
			Placebo	Therapy
Antiendotoxin[a]	4	2010	35%	35%
Antibody to interleukin-1 receptor	3	1898	35%	31%
Antibradykinin	2	755	36%	39%
AntiPAF	2	870	50%	45%
AntiTNF	8	4132	41%	40%
Soluble TNF receptor	2	688	38%	40%
NSAIDS	3	514	40%	37%
Steroids	9	1267	35%	39%
All studies	33	12034	38%	38%

Adapted from (Astiz and Rackow 1998). PAF, platelet-activating factor; TNF, tumor-necrosis factor alpha; NSAIDS, non-steroidal antiinflammatory drugs. [a] Antiendotoxin trials summarized here are those using anti-LPS core monoclonal antibodies or sera.

There are several explanations for these dissapointing findings. The first is that the populations of patients that have been enrolled in immunotherapeutic studies have been too small in each individual study to reliably exclude variations in disease severity, underlying conditions, pathogenicity of the microorganisms involved, and timing of inhibitor administration in the course of the septic process. It may have a quite different effect to infuse anti-TNFα in the early phase of sepsis compared to a later phase when interaction of this cytokine with target cells has occurred. The second is that gram-negative bacteria even when belonging to the same species may differ profoundly in their virulence. It has been shown in a mouse model of experimental peritonitis caused by a highly virulent E. coli strain that endogenous TNFα is needed for effective control of infection (Cross et al. 1989). In this model, a mouse strain was used that was unable to produce TNFα and IL-1 in response to endotoxin. Mice of this strain invariably succumbed to generalized peritonitis caused by this E. coli strain, while the same mice, when pretreated with TNFα and IL-1, were able to eliminate the bacteria. It must be emphasized that other E. coli strains exhibiting lesser virulence may affect the host not so much by their replication but by release of endotoxin, and inhibition of TNFα by monoclonal antibody may prove beneficial in this setting (Cross et al. 1989). Thus, TNFα may be both a beneficial and a harmful cytokine, but a critical level beyond which neutralization of this molecule makes sense has not been defined.

A third point to note is that the concept of human gram-negative sepsis that has formed the basis for the above-mentioned studies has now been recognized as being oversimplistic. In the past, it has been taken for granted that the pro-inflammatory cytokines such as TNFα, IL-1, IL-2, IL-12, IL-18 and interferon-γ are the major pathogenic molecules in the septic process. More recently, it has been

Fig. 9. Anti-inflammatory cytokine profile and mortality in febrile patients. In nearly all subgroups, patients with lethal infection had an elevated ratio of serum IL-10 to TNFα levels. Median IL-6 concentrations were also significantly higher in patients who died than in survivors (186 pg/ml *vs* 52 pg/ml, p < 0.001; data not shown). The study involved 464 patients (van Dissel et al. 1998)

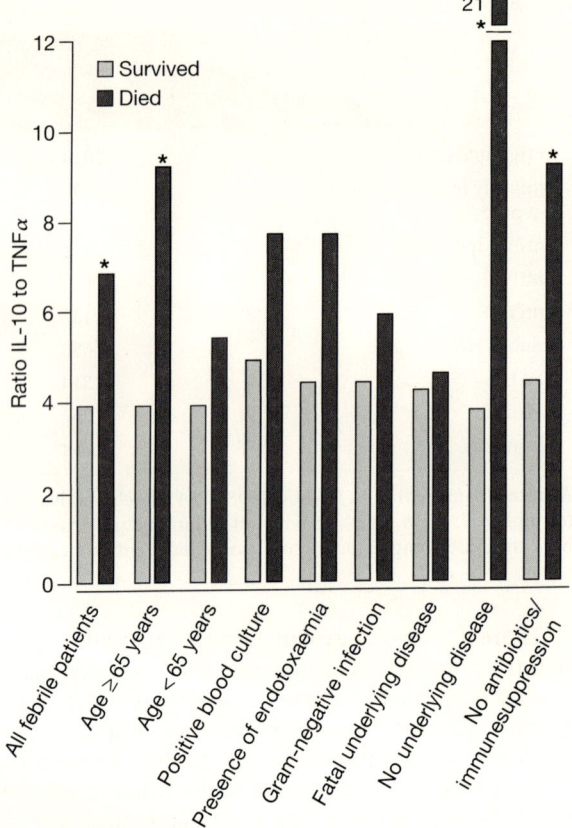

demonstrated that the host immune system counteracts these mediators quite early during the septic process by mounting an anti-inflammatory, compensatory response. The cytokines involved in this response have been identified as IL-4, IL-5, IL-6 and IL-10, and the septic syndrome in which these cytokines prevail has been called the compensatory anti-inflammatory response syndrome or CARS. It has been shown recently that the CARS syndrome, as characterized by an increased ratio of serum IL-10 to serum TNFα levels, develops in a significant number of febrile patients suffering from various kinds of infection, and that pronounced CARS correlates with increased mortality (Fig. 9) (van Dissel et al. 1998). This finding shows that many patients are able to generate antiinflammatory responses which may, however, be more detrimental than previously assumed. Therefore, the administration of anti-inflammatory agents of any kind may not be needed or may even be harmful.

Another aspect of CARS is a reduction of major histocompatibility complex class II HLA-DR expression on circulating monocytes. Levels of HLA-DR expression of less than 30% persisting for more than 2 days have been associated with a mortality of 58%, and persistence for more than 5 days with a mortality of 88%. Once monocyte inactivation is established in patients with sepsis, agents designed to minimize hyperinflammation are not likely to be effective (Kox et al. 1997). However, the administration of pro-inflammatory cytokines such as interferon-γ during this phase may also disturb the host's immunological balance and has been abandoned as a clinical option.

3.5.2
Factors and Mediators To Be Considered in Future Clinical Trials

From the above comments it becomes evident that the septic process following LPS binding to the monocyte is too complex to allow appropriate immunotherapeutic interventions. However, the early phase of LPS liberation (i.e. before endotoxin can bind to its target cells) appears to be worth further study. During this phase, several options exist which have been considered in the past and which may be clinically evaluated in the future. Agents such as the bactericidal permeability increasing protein (BPI), analogues of lipopolysaccharide binding protein (LBP) that are still able to bind endotoxin but have lost the ability to bind to CD14 (recombinant LBP analogues), soluble CD14, or monoclonal antibodies that bind to endotoxin may be useful. By contrast, neutralization of endotoxin by LPS-core-specific antibodies has failed to provide protection in clinical trials of both prophylaxis and therapy of gram-negative sepsis. Nevertheless, a short review of the history of this approach will be given here in order to facilitate the understanding while these attempts might have failed. The following paragraphs will also summarize the preliminary findings available for some of the newer anti-endotoxin agents.

Antisera or monoclonal antibodies to endotoxin core were first described by Chedid in the 1970s who proposed that such antibodies might occur naturally in humans and might act as an innate defense system against invading gram-negative pathogens (Chedid et al. 1968). Later studies by William McCabe, Abraham Braude and many other workers appeared at first to confirm this idea. The concept behind this was that all enterobacterial endotoxins share a common core structure composed of lipid A, ketodeoxyoctonic acid and a few oligosaccharide residues. Braude et al. raised antibodies against this structure by immunization of rabbits and showed protection against gram-negative sepsis in various animal models (for review, see (Cross et al. 1999)). Other authors, however, attempting to reproduce these findings, did not confirm a protective effect of core antiserum in animal models although the same immunization procedures were used (Greisman and Johnston 1988; Trautmann and Hahn 1985). Based on the promising experiences of Braude and coworkers, a human core LPS antiserum raised in volunteers was studied in a large clinical trial, and a significant protective effect could be shown (Ziegler et al. 1982). Later, monoclonal antibodies and hyperimmune globulins against the common core structure were developed and tested in clinical trials, however, the protective effects in terms of a reduction of sepsis mortality could never be as clearly reproduced as in the early animal experiments (Ziegler et al. 1991). Although the common core structure probably truely exists it is obviously not sufficiently exposed in intact gram-negative organisms or in intact free endotoxin to act as a binding site for passively administered antibodies (Mehra et al. 1993). Although some groups still pursue basic experimental studies of this concept (Bhattacharjee and Cross 1999), clinical applications will probably not be further pursued.

The *bactericidal/permeability-increasing protein* (BPI) is a 456-residue cationic protein produced only by precursors of polymorphonuclear leukocytes (PMN) and is stored in the primary granules of these cells. The potent cytotoxicity of BPI is limited to gram-negative bacteria, reflecting the extremely high affinity of BPI for endotoxin. The biological effects correlate with binding to LPS (Dahlberg et al. 1996). Interaction of BPI with live bacteria via LPS causes immediate growth arrest, followed by a damage to the inner membrane resulting in bacterial killing. Complex formation of BPI with cell-associated or cell-free LPS inhibits all LPS-induced host cell responses. BPI-blocking antibodies abolish the potent activity of whole PMN lysates and inflammatory fluids against BPI-sensitive gram-negative bacteria. The antibacterial and the anti-endotoxin activities of BPI are fully expressed by the amino terminal half of the molecule. These properties of BPI have prompted preclinical and subsequent clinical testing of recombinant amino-terminal fragments of BPI. In animals, human BPI derivatives protect against lethal injections of isolated LPS and challenge with gram-negative bacteria. Phase I trials in healthy human volunteers and multiple Phase I/II clinical trials have been completed or are in progress, and these trials among others also include severe peritoneal infections. Two phase III trials (meningococcemia and hemorrhagic trauma) have been initiated. Side effects in > 900 normal and severely ill individuals which have been treated so far have been minimal. Preliminary evidence points to an overall benefit in BPI-treated patients, but detailed results are not yet available because the products are protected by patents. As known so far, the results suggest that BPI may have a place in the treatment of life-threatening infections and conditions associated with bacteremia and endotoxemia (Elsbach 1998).

Polymyxin B is an agent with a binding site on LPS near to that or identical with that of BPI. It has been shown decades ago to be a potent LPS inactivating agent. Hemodialysis columns containing resins coated with polymyxin B have been used successfully in patients treated for lifethreatening septicemia, however, these anecdotal reports did not have further clinical implications. Systemic application of polymyxin B in sepsis is hampered by the considerable nephrotoxicity of this agent. However, recent studies have shown that the LPS-binding site of polymyxin B may be separated from the molecule and that synthetic compounds may be developed that retain the beneficial effects of polymyxin B but lack nephrotoxic effects (Iwagaka et al. 2000). Further studies in this direction appear promising.

The *lipopolysaccharide-binding protein (LPB)* is present in normal human serum and acts as a bridging molecule between LPS and the CD14 receptor on monocytes. If LPS binds first to LBP, its subsequent complex formation with CD14 occurs more rapidly and results in an early and strong inflammatory response. It was therefore tempting to develop analogues of LBP that are still able to bind endotoxin but do not have the capacity for bridging. Such recombinant molecules are currently under experimental study, but preparations suitable for human use have yet to be developed (Schuhmann 1992). It must be also noted that LBP, just like TNFα, has both beneficial and harmful effects. In highly virulent gram-negative organisms causing replicative infection, functionally active LBP seems to be required for control of infection (Jack et al. 1997).

The *CD14 receptor* itself is not a transmembranal molecule and therefore does not mediate LPS signals. Nevertheless, binding of LPS to CD14 is important for LPS recognition, and experimental studies in which the CD14 receptor was blocked by passively administered antibodies showed protection against LPS-induced shock and death (Leturcq et al. 1996). Recently, Frevert et al. demonstrated that this was also true in a model of bacteremic pneumonia established in rabbits. These authors noted that both neutralization of CD14 and antibacterial agents are necessary to combat established pulmonary infection because anti-CD14 by itself did not reduce the bacterial burden of the lung (Frevert et al. 2000). The significance of these findings for human infection has yet to be established. In surgical intensive care patients, high levels of soluble CD14 have been detected in the systemic circulation. Therefore, anti-CD14 antibodies might be captured by soluble CD14 in septic patients before reaching their target on the monocyte cell surface. Nevertheless, anti-CD14 may be another future option for immunotherapy of septic shock.

The *Toll-like receptor*, in particular Toll 4, is another molecule that appears to have a significant role for LPS binding to macrophages and, in particular, for the initiation of a functional macrophage response (Lien et al. 2000). However, little is known about the effects of blocking this receptor, and clinical antagonists have not yet been studied (Ingalls et al. 1999).

It is evident from this overview that a variety of potentially useful molecules are in the process of development, with some of them, such as the recombinant BPI products, being near to clinical introduction. It can be hoped that the high mortality of sepsis and septic shock caused by gram-negative organisms and their LPS may be lowered by such agents in the future. Patients suffering from secondary intraabdominal infections and peritoneal sepsis will be one of the major target groups for clinical trials of these agents.

3.5.3
Rationale for the Use of Intravenous Immunoglobulins

An immunotherapeutic approach that appears to act also through neutralization of endotoxin and other bacterial products is the passive administration of "normal" immunoglobulins derived from a large pool of healthy donors. At first sight, one could argue that septic patients also possess immunoglobulins in their sera and that it is unnecessary to supplement such antibodies during critical infections. However, a number of theoretical considerations and experimental findings support the concept that intravenous immunoglobulin (IVIG) may augment the host's immune defenses against both gram-negative and gram-positive bacteria.

The first consideration is that many patients suffer from a profound loss of immunoglobulins during critical disease and after surgery. When serial determinations of IgG and IgM serum levels were performed in patients after major surgery, a significant decrease of immunoglobulin serum concentrations was seen during the first week after the surgical intervention (Chitkara and Noronka 1977; Gauperaa et al. 1985). In some studies, the risk of postoperative infection correlated with reduced serum immunoglobulin concentrations. However, even if serum immunoglobulin concentrations are normal, there may be a lack of specific antibodies to pathogenic bacteria due consumption by binding to circulating endotoxin.

Secondly, a multitude of immunological studies have been performed to examine the spectrum of specific antibodies present in commercial immunoglobulin preparations. In a variety of studies, antibody concentrations against selected whole bacteria have been measured, and antibody titers have been given in arbitrary units such as twofold or tenfold dilution titers, or enzyme-linked immunosorbent assay (ELISA) units. A typical study was done by Hiemstra et al. who were able to show that six different commercial intravenous IgG products contained antibodies against whole cells of S. aureus, E. coli, Streptococcus pyogenes, B streptococci and pneumococci (Hiemstra et al. 1994). In another more recent study by Lamari et al., antibodies against a panel of gram-positive and gram-negative bacteria often encountered in ICUs were detected in two IVIG products (Lamari et al. 1999). It is not very useful, however, to know such titers or units because it has not been determined what titers are needed for effective antimicrobial defense in serum or tissue fluids. More recently, however, antibody determinations against surface molecules and exotoxins of gram-positive bacteria have been performed which included sera from diseased and healthy individuals as controls. In these studies, it was shown that commercial IVIGs possess antibodies against streptococcal M proteins (Basma et al. 1998), streptococcal pyrogenic exotoxins A and B (Mascini et al. 1999; Norrby-Teglund et al. 1998), or – in an earlier study – staphylococcal toxic shock syndrome toxin-1 (Dickgiesser and Kustermann 1996). When compared with the sera of individuals suffering from streptococcal or staphylococcal toxic shock, it became apparent that diseased individuals had very low levels of antibody against the exotoxin associated with their infection, and that levels of anti-exotoxin antibody in IVIG exceeded such levels by factors of up to ten (Mascini et al. 1999). Therefore, it appeared logical to administer IVIG at high doses to patients with bacterial toxic shock syndrome, and significant protection has been recently shown in 21 patients with streptococcal toxic shock who were compared with 32 historical controls (Kaul et al. 1999). The mitogenic activity induced by the pyrogenic exotoxins involved in these cases was inhibited significantly by post-infusion patient sera, while this was the case for only a minor portion of patients prior to infusion of IVIG (Kaul et al. 1999). Similar findings in a group of 15 patients compared with historical controls had been reported previously (Norrby and Norrby-Tegtlund 1997).

The amount of antibody against endotoxins of gram-negative bacteria has recently been examined by our own group in a panel of commercially available IVIG preparations. For this study, we first determined which endotoxin or LPS serotypes are commonly associated with gram-negative septicemia in the clinical setting. Escherichia coli, Klebsiella spp. and Pseudomonas aeruginosa are known to be the gram-negative organisms most frequently involved in nosocomial septicemia. However, these bacterial species exhibit a variety of different LPS serotypes. A literature review revealed, that for E. coli, the LPS (O serotype) antigens most frequently detected in septicemia were O1, O2, O4, O6, O15, O16 and O18 and O75 which together account for > 80 % of the antigenic types. For Klebsiella, our own group showed that the O antigen serogroups O1, O2ab and O3 were found in 79.8 % of bacteremic isolates. Finally, for Pseudomonas aeruginosa, various studies were available which indicated that the Fisher-Devlin O serotypes FD 1–5 were predominant in the setting of clinical sepsis. Using reference organisms for these antigens judged to be important, we purified their

Fig. 10. Antibody levels against gram-negative bacterial LPS in commercial IVIG preparations as determined by quantitative ELISA. **A,** IgG antibody levels measured in Sandoglobulin® (2 batches) and Pentaglobin® (4 batches). **B,** IgM antibody levels measured in Pentaglobin® (4 batches)

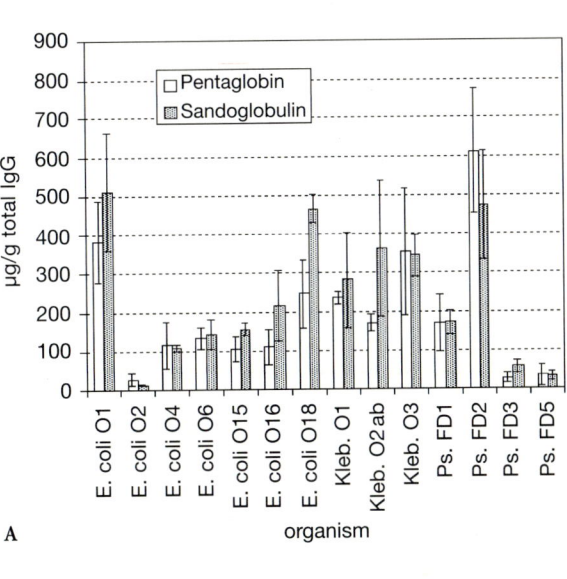

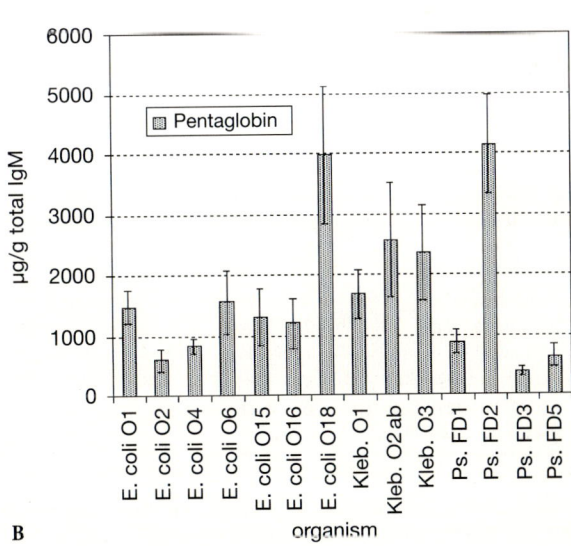

LPSs and used these preparations for the study of the anti-endotoxin antibody content of immunoglobulin preparations. As controls, a rough E. coli LPS derived from E. coli J5, and LPS from Vibrio cholerae was used. The latter preparation was chosen because it was anticipated that sera of mid-European or North-American donors whould not harbor antibodies against Vibrio cholerae. Both a quantitative ELISA system yielding gravimetric antibody concentration values, and Western blotting as a means to study the specificity of antibodies were applied (Trautmann et al. 1998).

In this study, we found a relatively high batch uniformity among different lots of IVIG studied. All products contained measurable antibody levels against smooth LPSs of the organisms studied. Mean total antibody levels, expressed in μg per ml of final product, were highest in one of three IVIG products containing IgG only, and in a product containing both IgG and IgM as well as IgA. Virtually no antibodies were detected against rough mutant LPS and LPS from Vibrio cholerae, indicating that the natural antibodies contained in these products are directed against „smooth" determinants of organisms commonly encountered in industrialized countries. The relative distribution of O antigen antibody levels against different LPS serotypes in these products is depicted in Fig. 10.

When examining in more detail the role of IgM in this context, we found that the only available product enriched in IgM (Pentaglobin®) exhibited remarkably high antibody concentrations in its IgM fraction. Table 9 shows the mean antibody levels against each O antigen studied, expressed as μg per g of total immunoglobulin of the respective class. It is evident from these data that endotoxin antibodies are apparently concentrated in human IgM, a finding that confirms earlier observations that "natural" antibodies are those of the IgM class.

Table 9. LPS-specific IgG and IgM antibody content in four batches of a commercial IgG/A/M preparation

LPS antigen	Specific IgG (mean ± SD) [μg/g total IgG]	Specific IgM (mean ± SD) [μg/g total IgM]	Fold difference
E. coli O1	383 ± 122	1481 ± 274	3.9
E. coli O2	28 ± 19	595 ± 217	21.3
E. coli O4	115 ± 68	821 ± 139	7.1
E. coli O6	135 ± 33	1555 ± 614	11.5
E. coli O15	106 ± 38	1295 ± 543	12.2
E. coli O16	111 ± 53	1198 ± 480	10.8
E. coli O18	247 ± 102	3985 ± 1313	16.1
Klebsiella O1	237 ± 19	1676 ± 464	7.1
Klebsiella O2ab	170 ± 24	2566 ± 1084	15.1
Klebsiella O3	355 ± 190	2351 ± 912	6.6
Pseudomonas FD1	170 ± 85	877 ± 230	5.2
Pseudomonas FD2	613 ± 184	4146 ± 938	6.8
Pseudomonas FD3	28 ± 13	378 ± 84	13.5
Pseudomonas FD5	35 ± 31	638 ± 214	18.2

Adapted from (Trautmann et al. 1998). SD, standard deviation; FD, Fisher-Devlin serotype. Fold differences were calculated from mean values.

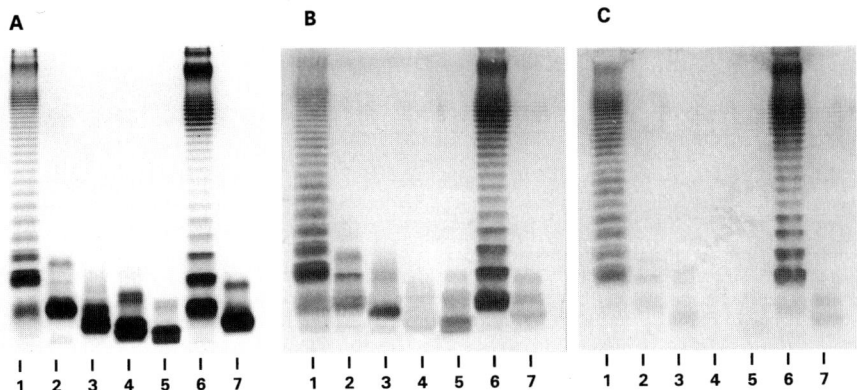

Fig. 11. Immunoblotting experiment demonstrating the presence of LPS-specific antibodies in IgG and IgM of commercial IVIG products. Lane 1, Salmonella minnesota wild-type LPS; lanes 2–5, Salmonella Ra, Rc, Rd and Re chemotype LPS; lane 6, E. coli O18 smooth LPS; lane 7, E. coli J5 LPS. **A**, silver-stained gel; **B**, immunoblot reacted with Sandoglobulin, **C**, immunoblot reacted with IgM purified from Pentaglobin

In order to roughly determine the epitope specificity of the antibodies found in these products, we performed Western blot experiments in which the LPS antigens were separated by gel electrophoresis, and the IgG and IgG/A/M products used as primary binding antibodies. Figure 11 shows a representative experiment. The IgG product tested contained antibodies both against smooth E. coli and Salmonella LPS as well as antibodies to rough LPS. The latter finding was somewhat discrepant to the ELISA data, but may be explained by the higher sensitivity of Western blotting for detecting antibodies. The IgM product contained antibodies mainly directed against smooth LPS determinants.

In a separate set of experiments, we asked whether such LPS-specific antibodies would show functional activity in terms of neutralizing LPS-mediated effects. Using an in vitro cell culture system, we challenged human macrophages with LPS, which stimulated the cells to secrete human TNFα into the culture supernatant. When various IVIGs were added to the cell culture medium together with LPS, the amount of TNFα released was reduced by up to 70%. The commercial products Pentaglobin® and Polyglobin N® showed the highest inhibitory effect in this system which corresponded to their high antibody levels against the LPSs used (Table 10).

While all of these data were generated by in vitro experiments, it must be asked whether the concentrations of LPS-specific antibodies in IVIG products will be sufficient to treat human gram-negative septicemia. Few data are available from humans which correlate effective protection against clinical infection with humoral antibody levels. For pneumococcal infection, it has been shown that antibody levels > 1 µg/ml against individual serotype polysaccharide antigens correlate with protection against systemic disease. Similarly, for invasive H. influenzae infections, antibody levels > 0.1 µg/ml have been shown to be protective. It is not known which level of antibody is needed for successful control of gram-negative septicemia in humans. To our knowledge, Schiff et al. performed

Table 10. Inhibition of LPS-induced TNF release by IVIGs

Product	% Inhibition (mean ± SD) versus control		
	E. coli O18	Klebsiella O1	Pseudomonas FD1
Pentaglobin	27.5 ± 14.5	62.5 ± 15.2	45.0 ± 11.4
Sandoglobulin	22.4 ± 17.2	42.0 ± 15.4	27.1 ± 21.6
Intraglobin F	24.8 ± 17.3	54.5 ± 14.4	36.9 ± 9.0
Polyglobin N	36.5 ± 4.0	72.1 ± 17.6	38.6 ± 9.4
HBsAG mAb	none	none	none
no. of expts.	4	6	6

From (Trautmann et al. 1997).

the only experimental study of gram-negative bacteremia in a rat model of E. coli
(O serotype 18) infection in which protective serum levels of O-antigen specific
LPS immunoglobulin were estimated (Schiff et al. 1993). In this study, animals
were pretreated with rabbit or human hyperimmune IgG at increasing doses and
then left resting for 24 hours. The next day, serum levels of specific IgG were
determined by ELISA, and the animals challenged with live E. coli bacteria at
otherwise lethal doses. The relationship between anti-O18 LPS IgG levels at
disease onset (expressed in µg/ml of serum) and the development of bacteremia
is shown in Fig. 12. It was concluded by these authors that a concentration of
~ 1 µg/ml of circulating antibody protected against bacteremia. In another series

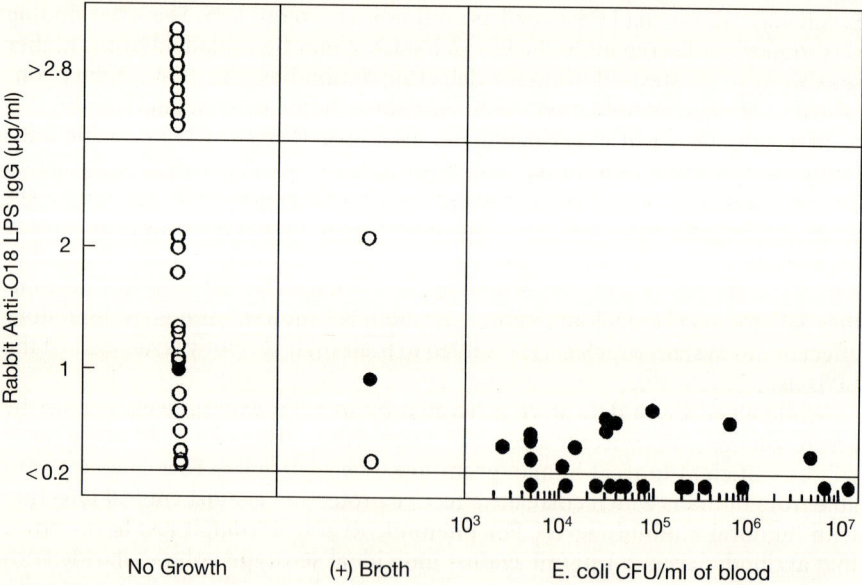

Fig. 12. Relationship between intensity of bacteremia and LPS-specific antibody levels at disease
onset in a model of E. coli septicemia in rats. Bacteremia did virtually not occur in the presence
of antibody levels > 1 µg/ml (Schiff et al. 1993). Black dots (•) denote decreased animals, whereas circles (○) characterize surviving rats. No growth marks negative cultures; (+) Broth indicates
positive broth

Table 11. Protective effect of human anti-O18 LPS IgG against bacteremic E. coli infection in rats

Treatment (no. of animals)	No. of animals with bacteremia (%)	No. of deaths (%)	geometric mean anti-O18 LPS serum level (µg/ml ± SD)
Human anti-O18 LPS IgG			
2.4 µg (14)	1 (7)	3 (21)	2.6 ± 1.9
1.2 µg	2 (22)	1 (11)	1.2 ± 0.06
0.1 µg	2 (100)	1 (50)	0.04 ± 0.005
Preimmune human IgG (4)	4 (100)	4 (100)	0.02 ± 0.01
Saline (7)	7 (100)	7 (100)	0.02 ± 0.02

From (Schiff et al. 1993).

of experiments, the authors pretreated the animals with human anti-O18 IgG and recorded both bacteremia and mortality. Again, 1 µg/ml appeared to be the level of specific serum antibody needed to confer protection (Table 11).

How can these experimental figures be translated into immunoglobulin doses needed in human IVIG therapy for gram-negative septicemia? Our own quantitative studies have shown that commercial IgG preparations contain between 30 and 600 µg specific antibody per gram of total IgG (cf. Table 9). Given an adult human blood volume of about 5 Liter, and a target concentration of specific antibody of ~ 1 µg/ml (corresponding to 1 mg/L), it can be calculated that the total dose of specific antibody that needs to be infused is about 5 mg. If a concentration of specific antibody of at least 100 µg/g (0.1 mg/g) of total IgG is accepted as being available for most pathogens, one would need to infuse 50 g of immunoglobulin peparation. Most products have a 5 % concentration of IgG, and therefore the volume to be infused would be 1000 ml. This could be done by infusing 300–400 ml per day on three consecutive days. Although these calculations depend on a number of variables that have been documented each in only a single study (namely that the target antibody level is ~ 1µg/ml and that > 100 µg/g is available in IVIG), it appears interesting that in studies, in which high doses of IVIG exceeding 50 g were infused, beneficial effects were demonstrated, while failures occurred more often in studies with much lower IVIG doses. For instance, in the study by Dominioni et al., a total of 60 g of IgG were infused, and mortality rates were 67 % in 33 control patients and 38 % in 29 IVIG-treated patients (Dominioni et al. 1991). Beneficial findings were also reported from a large multicenter trial performed in which large doses of 40–60 g of IVIG were used (Prophylactic intravenous administration of … 1992). By contrast, other authors, using relatively low doses, did not see beneficial effects (for review, see (Nydegger 1997)).

Due to the relatively high amount of specific antibodies contained in the IgM fraction of human plasma, a product enriched in IgM might need lesser doses to afford protection, however, dose-response studies are not available for this product. In general, 20 g of this product have been found to be effective (Just et al. 1986; Schedel et al. 1991).

It is beyond the scope of this chapter to review the tremendous amount of clinical literature that has been devoted to the use of IVIG in the clinical setting.

The reader is referred to the recent meta-analysis performed by the Cochrane Infectious Diseases Group which included 23 out of 49 prospective randomized clinical studies that fulfilled their critical inclusion criteria. In this analysis the authors found a significant benefit of IVIG used for the treatment of adult septic patients. Most studies had been done with surgical patients. It was interesting to note – and compatible with our in vitro findings – that among the polyclonal IVIG trials, those using IgM-enriched immunoglobulins demonstrated a greater benefit (Alejandria et al. 2000). The authors suggested that larger clinical trials should be performed and that, in future trials, a number of variables should be more clearly defined. For instance, the clinical definition of sepsis should be refined, patients should be stratified for underlying diseases and severity of sepsis, and other end points than mortality should be examined, e.g. the reversal of organ failure (Alejandria et al. 2000). Pending those studies, the results of the Cochrane analysis speak in favour of the use if IVIGs for critical septic patients in intensive care.

Literature

Prophylactic intravenous administration of standard immune globulin as compared with core-lipopolysaccharide immune globulin in patients at high risk of postsurgical infection. The Intravenous Immunoglobulin Collaborative Study Group (1992) N Engl J Med 327(4): 234–240

Aldridge KE, Ashcraft DS (1997) Comparison of the in vitro activities of Bay 12-8039, a new quinolone, and other antimicrobials against clinically important anaerobes. Antimicrob Agents Chemother 41(3): 709–711

Alejandria MM, Lansang MA, Dans LF, Mantaring JB (2000) Intravenous immunoglobulin for treating sepsis and septic shock. Cochrane Database Syst Rev (2): CD001090

Ariza J, Gudiol F, Dolz C, Xiol J, Linares J, Bosch J, Pallares R (1986) Evaluation of aztreonam in the treatment of spontaneous bacterial peritonitis in patients with cirrhosis. Hepatology 6(5): 906–910

Astiz ME, Rackow EC (1998) Septic shock. Lancet 351(9114): 1501–1505

Basma H, Norrby-Teglund A, McGeer A, Low DE, El-Ahmedy O, Dale JB, Schwartz B, Kotb M (1998) Opsonic antibodies to the surface M protein of group A streptococci in pooled normal immunoglobulins (IVIG): potential impact on the clinical efficacy of IVIG therapy for severe invasive group A streptococcal infections. Infect Immun 66(5): 2279–2283

Bassi C, Falconi M, Talamini G, Uomo G, Papaccio G, Dervenis C, Salvia R, Minelli EB, Pederzoli P (1998) Controlled clinical trial of pefloxacin versus imipenem in severe acute pancreatitis. Gastroenterology 115(6): 1513–1517

Bassi C, Pederzoli P, Vesentini S, Falconi M, Bonora A, Abbas H, Benini A, Bertazzoni EM (1994) Behavior of antibiotics during human necrotizing pancreatitis. Antimicrob Agents Chemother 38(4): 830–836

Beger HG, Bittner R, Block S, Buchler M (1986) Bacterial contamination of pancreatic necrosis. A prospective clinical study. Gastroenterology 91(2): 433–438

Bhattacharjee AK, Cross AS (1999) Vaccines and antibodies in the prevention and treatment of sepsis. Infect Dis Clin North Am 13(2): 355–369, vii

Billing A, Frohlich D, Ruckdeschel G (1992) The effect of taurolin on endogenous immunity and pathogen elimination in human peritonitis. Langenbecks Arch Chir 377(3): 180–185

Blot F, Nitenberg G, Chachaty E, Raynard B, Germann N, Antoun S, Laplanche A, Brun-Buisson C, Tancrede C (1999) Diagnosis of catheter-related bacteraemia: a prospective comparison of the time to positivity of hub-blood versus peripheral-blood cultures. Lancet 354(9184): 1071–1077

Bongaerts G, Roelofs-Willemse H (1998) In vitro expression of beta-lactam-induced response by clinical gram- negative bacteria with the potential for inducible beta-lactamase production. Scand J Infect Dis 30(6): 579–583

Bryant RE, Mazza JA (1989) Effect of the abscess environment on the antimicrobial activity of ciprofloxacin. Am J Med 87(5A): 23S–27S

Buchler M, Malfertheiner P, Friess H, Isenmann R, Vanek E, Grimm H, Schlegel P, Friess T, Beger HG (1992) Human pancreatic tissue concentration of bactericidal antibiotics. Gastroenterology 103(6): 1902–1908

Chedid L, Parant M, Parant F, Boyer F (1968) A proposed mechanism for natural immunity to enterobacterial pathogens. J Immunol 100(2): 292–306

Chien JW, Kucia ML, Salata RA (2000) Use of linezolid, an oxazolidinone, in the treatment of multidrug- resistant gram-positive bacterial infections. Clin Infect Dis 30(1): 146–151

Chitkara YK, Noronha AB (1977) Serum immunoglobulins after surgical operations. Int Surg 62(3): 165–168

Cockerill FR, Hughes JG, Vetter EA, Mueller RA, Weaver AL, Ilstrup DM, Rosenblatt JE, Wilson WR (1997) Analysis of 281,797 consecutive blood cultures performed over an eight- year period: trends in microorganisms isolated and the value of anaerobic culture of blood. Clin Infect Dis 24(3): 403–418

Collins MD, Dajani AS, Kim KS, King DR, Kaplan SL, Azimi PH, Kolokathis A, Swanson R (1998) Comparison of ampicillin/sulbactam plus aminoglycoside vs. ampicillin plus clindamycin plus aminoglycoside in the treatment of intraabdominal infections in children. The Multicenter Group. Pediatr Infect Dis J 17(3 Suppl): S15–S18

Cross AS, Opal SM, Bhattacharjee K, Donta ST, Peduzzi PN, Furer E, Que JU, Cryz SJ (1999) Immunotherapy of sepsis: flawed concept or faulty implementation? Vaccine 17 Suppl 2: S13–S21

Cross AS, Sadoff JC, Kelly N, Bernton E, Gemski P (1989) Pretreatment with recombinant murine tumor necrosis factor alpha/cachectin and murine interleukin 1 alpha protects mice from lethal bacterial infection. J Exp Med 169(6): 2021–2027

Csendes A, Burdiles P, Maluenda F, Diaz JC, Csendes P, Mitru N (1996) Simultaneous bacteriologic assessment of bile from gallbladder and common bile duct in control subjects and patients with gallstones and common duct stones. Arch Surg 131(4): 389–394

Dahlberg PS, Acton RD, Battafarano RJ, Uknis ME, Ratz CA, Johnston JW, Haseman JR, Gray BH, Dunn DL (1996) A novel endotoxin antagonist attenuates tumor necrosis factor-alpha secretion. J Surg Res 63(1): 44–48

Dickgiesser N, Kustermann B (1986) IgG antibodies against toxic shock syndrome toxin 1 in human immunoglobulins. Klin Wochenschr 64(14): 633–635

Dominioni L, Dionigi R, Zanello M, Chiaranda M, Acquarolo A, Ballabio A, Sguotti C (1991) Effects of high-dose IgG on survival of surgical patients with sepsis scores of 20 or greater. Arch Surg 126(2): 236–240

Elsbach P (1998) The bactericidal/permeability-increasing protein (BPI) in antibacterial host defense. J Leukoc Biol 64(1): 14–18

Frevert CW, Matute-Bello G, Skerrett SJ, Goodman RB, Kajikawa O, Sittipunt C, Martin TR (2000) Effect of CD14 blockade in rabbits with Escherichia coli pneumonia and sepsis. J Immunol 164(10): 5439–5445

Fugger R, Hamilton G, Rogy M, Herbst F, Kwasny W, Schemper M, Schultz F (1990) Prognostic significance of endotoxin determination in patients with severe intraabdominal infection. J Infect Dis 161(6): 1314–1315

Gauperaa T, Giercksky KE, Revhaug A, Rekvig OP (1985) Fibronectin, complement and immunoglobulins in serum after surgery. Br J Surg 72(1): 59–62

Gilbert DN, Moellering RC, Sande MA (1999) 59. Hyde Park, Vermont, USA, Antimicrobial Therapy Inc. The Sanford guide to antimicrobial therapy

Gorenstein A, Gewurtz G, Serour F, Somekh E (1994) Postappendectomy intra-abdominal abscess: a therapeutic approach. Arch Dis Child 70(5): 400–402

Grange JD, Amiot X, Grange V, Gutmann L, Biour M, Bodin F, Poupon R (1990) Amoxicillin-clavulanic acid therapy of spontaneous bacterial peritonitis: a prospective study of twenty-seven cases in cirrhotic patients. Hepatology 11(3): 360–364

Greisman SE, Johnston CA (1988) Failure of antisera to J5 and R595 rough mutants to reduce endotoxemic lethality. J Infect Dis 157(1): 54–64

Hiemstra PS, Brands-Tajouiti J, van Furth R (1994) Comparison of antibody activity against various microorganisms in intravenous immunoglobulin preparations determined by ELISA and opsonic assay. J Lab Clin Med 123(2): 241–246

Hoogkamp-Korstanje JA (1995) Ciprofloxacin vs. cefotaxime regimens for the treatment of intra-abdominal infections. Infection 23(5): 278–282

Ingalls RR, Heine H, Lien E, Yoshimura A, Golenbock D (1999) Lipopolysaccharide recognition, CD14, and lipopolysaccharide receptors. Infect Dis Clin North Am 13(2): 341–253, vii

Isenmann R, Friess H, Schlegel P, Fleischer K, Buchler MW (1994) Penetration of ciprofloxacin into the human pancreas. Infection 22(5): 343–346

Iwagaki A, Porro M, Pollack M (2000) Influence of synthetic antiendotoxin peptides on lipopolysaccharide (LPS) recognition and LPS-induced proinflammatory cytokine responses by cells expressing membrane-bound CD14. Infect Immun 68(3): 1655–1663

Jack RS, Fan X, Bernheiden M, Rune G, Ehlers M, Weber A, Kirsch G, Mentel R, Furll B, Freudenberg M et al. (1997) Lipopolysaccharide-binding protein is required to combat a murine gram-negative bacterial infection. Nature 389(6652): 742–745

Javid G, Khan BA, Shah AH, Gulzar GM, Khan MA (1998) Short-course ceftriaxone therapy in spontaneous bacterial peritonitis. Postgrad Med J 74(876): 592–595

Just HM, Metzger M, Vogel W, Pelka RB (1986) Effect of adjuvant immunoglobulin therapy on infections in patients in an surgical intensive care unit. Results of a randomized controlled study. Klin Wochenschr 64(6): 245–256

Kanellakopoulou K, Giamarellou H, Papadothomakos P, Tsipras H, Chloroyiannis J, Theakou R, Sfikakis P (1993) Meropenem versus imipenem/cilastatin in the treatment of intraabdominal infections requiring surgery. Eur J Clin Microbiol Infect Dis 12(6): 449–453

Kaul R, McGeer A, Norrby-Teglund A, Kotb M, Schwartz B, O'Rourke K, Talbot J, Low DE (1999) Intravenous immunoglobulin therapy for streptococcal toxic shock syndrome – a comparative observational study. The Canadian Streptococcal Study Group. Clin Infect Dis 28(4): 800–807

Kolbert CP, Persing DH (1999) Ribosomal DNA sequencing as a tool for identification of bacterial pathogens. Curr Opin Microbiol 2(3): 299–305

Konig C, Simmen HP, Blaser J (1998) Bacterial concentrations in pus and infected peritoneal fluid – implications for bactericidal activity of antibiotics. J Antimicrob Chemother 42(2): 227–232

Kox WJ, Bone RC, Krausch D, Docke WD, Kox SN, Wauer H, Egerer K, Querner S, Asadullah K, von Baehr R et al (1997) Interferon gamma-1b in the treatment of compensatory anti-inflammatory response syndrome. A new approach: proof of principle. Arch Intern Med 157(4): 389–393

Lamari F, Anastassiou ED, Tsegenidis T, Dimitracopoulos G, Karamanos NK (1999) An enzyme immunoassay to determine the levels of specific antibodies toward bacterial surface antigens in human immunoglobulin preparations and blood serum. J Pharm Biomed Anal 20(6): 913–920

Leturcq DJ, Moriarty AM, Talbott G, Winn RK, Martin TR, Ulevitch RJ (1996) Antibodies against CD14 protect primates from endotoxin-induced shock. J Clin Invest 98(7): 1533–1538

Levin J, Poore TE, Zauber NP, Oser RS (1970) Detection of endotoxin in the blood of patients with sepsis due to gram-negative bacteria. N Engl J Med 283(24): 1313–1316

Li J, Plorde JJ, Carlson LG (1994) Effects of volume and periodicity on blood cultures. J Clin Microbiol 32(11): 2829–2831

Lien E, Means TK, Heine H, Yoshimura A, Kusumoto S, Fukase K, Fenton MJ, Oikawa M, Qureshi N, Monks B et al (2000) Toll-like receptor 4 imparts ligand-specific recognition of bacterial lipopolysaccharide. J Clin Invest 105(4): 497–504

Livermore DM (1987) Clinical significance of beta-lactamase induction and stable derepression in gram-negative rods. Eur J Clin Microbiol 6(4): 439–445

Mascini EM, Jansze M, Verhoef J, van Dijk H (1999) Relative avidities of human immunoglobulin G antibodies for streptococcal pyrogenic exotoxins A and B. Clin Diagn Lab Immunol 6(6): 977–980

Mehra IV, Gottlieb JE, Nash DB (1993) Monoclonal antibody therapy for gram-negative sepsis: principles, applications, and controversies. Pharmacotherapy 13(2): 128–134

Midy D, Pometan JP, Baste JC, Pajadon V (1992) Study of the efficacy and tolerance of imipenem-cilastatin used as monotherapy for the adjuvant treatment to surgery of peritonitis. Results of a French multicenter study including 257 patients. J Chir (Paris)129(6–7): 303–308

Mock CN, Jurkovich GJ, Dries DJ, Maier RV (1995) Clinical significance of antibiotic endotoxin-releasing properties in trauma patients. Arch Surg 130(11): 1234–1240

Norrby-Teglund A, Basma H, Andersson J, McGeer A, Low DE, Kotb M (1998) Varying titers of neutralizing antibodies to streptococcal superantigens in different preparations of normal polyspecific immunoglobulin G: implications for therapeutic efficacy [see comments]. Clin Infect Dis 26(3): 631–638

Norrby SR, Norrby-Tegtlund A (1997) Infections due to group A streptococcus: new concepts and potential treatment strategies. Annals of the Academy of Medicine of Singapore 26, 691–693

Nydegger UE (1997) Sepsis and polyspecific intravenous immunoglobulins. J Clin Apheresis 12(2): 93–99

Ohlin B, Cederberg A, Forssell H, Solhaug JH, Tveit E (1999) Piperacillin/tazobactam compared with cefuroxime/ metronidazole in the treatment of intra-abdominal infections. Eur J Surg 165(9): 875–884

Prins JM, van Agtmael MA, Kuijper EJ, van Deventer SJ, Speelman P (1995) Antibiotic-induced endotoxin release in patients with gram-negative urosepsis: a double-blind study comparing imipenem and ceftazidime. J Infect Dis 172(3): 886–891

Reetze-Bonorden P, Bohler J, Keller E (1993) Drug dosage in patients during continuous renal replacement therapy. Pharmacokinetic and therapeutic considerations. Clin Pharmacokinet 24(5): 362–379

Rosman C, Westerveld GJ, Kooi K, Bleichrodt RP (1999) Local treatment of generalised peritonitis in rats; effects on bacteria, endotoxin and mortality. Eur J Surg 165(11): 1072–1079

Ruhnke M, Schmidt-Westhausen A, Engelmann E, Trautmann M (1996) Comparative evaluation of three antifungal susceptibility test methods for Candida albicans isolates and correlation with response to fluconazole therapy. J Clin Microbiol 34(12): 3208–3011

Ruhnke M, Yeates RA, Pfaff G, Sarnow E, Hartmann A, Trautmann M (1995) Single-dose pharmacokinetics of fluconazole in patients with liver cirrhosis. J Antimicrob Chemother 35(5): 641–647

Runyon BA, Akriviadis EA, Sattler FR, Cohen J (1991) Ascitic fluid and serum cefotaxime and desacetyl cefotaxime levels in patients treated for bacterial peritonitis. Dig Dis Sci 36(12): 1782–1786

Runyon BA, McHutchison JG, Antillon MR, Akriviadis EA, Montano AA (1991) Short-course ver sus long-course antibiotic treatment of spontaneous bacterial peritonitis. A randomized controlled study of 100 patients. Gastroenterology 100(6): 1737–1742

Schedel I, Dreikhausen U, Nentwig B, Hockenschnieder M, Rauthmann D, Balikcioglu S, Coldewey R, Deicher H (1991) Treatment of gram-negative septic shock with an immunoglobulin preparation: a prospective, randomized clinical trial. Crit Care Med 19(9): 1104–1113

Schiff DE, Wass CA, Cryz SJJ, Cross AS, Kim KS (1993) Estimation of protective levels of anti-O-specific lipopolysaccharide immunoglobulin G antibody against experimental Escherichia coli infection. Infect Immun 61(3): 975–980

Schoeffel U, Jacobs E, Ruf G, Mierswa F, von Specht BU, Farthmann EH (1995) Intraperitoneal micro-organisms and the severity of peritonitis. Eur J Surg 161(7): 501–508

Schumann RR (1992) Function of lipopolysaccharide (LPS)-binding protein (LBP) and CD14, the receptor for LPS/LBP complexes: a short review. Res Immunol 143(1): 11–15

Shenep JL, Barton RP, Mogan KA (1985) Role of antibiotic class in the rate of liberation of endotoxin during therapy for experimental gram-negative bacterial sepsis. J Infect Dis 151(6): 1012–1018

Simpson AJ, Opal SM, Angus BJ, Prins JM, Palardy JE, Parejo NA, Chaowagul W, White NJ (2000) Differential antibiotic-induced endotoxin release in severe melioidosis. J Infect Dis 181(3): 1014–1019

Spitalnic SJ, Woolard RH, Mermel LA (1995) The significance of changing needles when inoculating blood cultures: a meta-analysis. Clin Infect Dis 21(5): 1103–1106

Trautmann M, Hahn H (1985) Antiserum against Escherichia coli J5: a re-evaluation of its in vitro and in vivo activity against heterologous gram-negative bacteria. Infection 13(3): 140–145

Trautmann M, Heinemann M, Moricke A, Seidelmann M, Lorenz I, Berger D, Steinbach G, Schneider M (1999) Endotoxin release due to ciprofloxacin measured by three different methods. J Chemother11(4): 248–254

Trautmann M, Held TK, Susa M, Karajan MA, Wulf A, Cross AS, Marre R (1998) Bacterial lipopolysaccharide (LPS)-specific antibodies in commercial human immunoglobulin preparations: superior antibody content of an IgM- enriched product. Clin Exp Immunol 111(1): 81–90

Trautmann M, Karajan MA, Susa M, Marre R, Gansauge F (1997) Intravenous immunoglobulins inhibit LPS-induced TNFalpha release from human monocytic cells. Faist E, editor. Congress proceedings, 4th International Congress on the Immune Consequences of Trauma, Shock and Sepsis. 775–779. Bologna, Italy, Monduzzi

van Dissel JT, van Langevelde P, Westendorp RG, Kwappenberg K, Frolich M (1998) Anti-inflammatory cytokine profile and mortality in febrile patients. Lancet 351(9107): 950–953

Washington JA (1975) Blood cultures: principles and techniques. Mayo Clin Proc 50(2): 91–98

Weinstein MP (1996) Current blood culture methods and systems: clinical concepts, technology, and interpretation of results. Clin Infect Dis 23(1): 40–46

Weinstein MP, Reller LB, Murphy JR, Lichtenstein KA (1983) The clinical significance of positive blood cultures: a comprehensive analysis of 500 episodes of bacteremia and fungemia in adults. I. Laboratory and epidemiologic observations. Rev Infect Dis 5(1): 35–53

Wendt C, Krause C, Xander LU, Loffler D, Floss H (1999) Prevalence of colonization with vancomycin-resistant enterococci in various population groups in Berlin, Germany. J Hosp Infect 42(3): 193–200

Wittmann DH, Welter J, Schassan HH (1982) Antibiotic concentrations in the abdominal cavity as basis for antibacterial therapy of peritonitis: penetration of mezlocillin into the peritoneal exudate. Infection 10 Suppl 3: S204–S208

Ziegler EJ, Fisher CJJ, Sprung CL, Straube RC, Sadoff JC, Foulke GE, Wortel CH, Fink MP, Dellinger RP, Teng NN (1991) Treatment of gram-negative bacteremia and septic shock with HA-1A human monoclonal antibody against endotoxin. A randomized, double-blind, placebo-controlled trial. The HA-1A Sepsis Study Group. N Engl J Med 324(7): 429–436

Ziegler EJ, McCutchan JA, Fierer J, Glauser MP, Sadoff JC, Douglas H, Braude AI (1982) Treatment of gram-negative bacteremia and shock with human antiserum to a mutant Escherichia coli. N Engl J Med 307(20): 1225–1230

Intensive Care Management in Abdominal Surgical Patients with Septic Complications

E. HANISCH and A. ENCKE

4.1
Epidemiology and Outcome of SIRS, Sepsis and Septic Shock

The pathology of sepsis shows an increasing incidence. The reasons for this fact are an increased life expectancy in the total population, the clear rise in the survival time of chronically ill patients, the relative frequency of sepsis with AIDS, the increasing number of antibiotic therapies, the administration of glucocorticoids, the use of mechanical implants and the improved possibilities of artificial ventilation.

Definitions of sepsis as an independent syndrome vary not only in the relevant literature but also in clinical practice. In 1914 Schottmüller (Schottmüller 1914) gave a pathogenic definition of sepsis that said "A sepsis is given when a focus has formed within the body from which pathogenic bacteria are continually or periodically released into the blood circulation and it is in this way that this invasion causes subjective and objective symptoms."

To improve research on sepsis, standardised definitions are required for the terms of infection, bacteraemia, sepsis and septic shock. As a result, comparable groups of patients could allow the comparative and objective assessment of new therapies. In 1991 a "Consensus Conference" (ACCP/CCM), held in Northbrook (USA) (Bone et al. 1992), took into account these efforts by defining the terms of infection, bacteraemia, SIRS (Systemic Inflammatory Response Syndrome), sepsis, severe sepsis, septic shock, and MODS (Multiple Organ Dysfunction Syndrome).

In the following, the terms of the Consensus Conference (SIRS, sepsis and septic shock) will be applied to intensive care patients of a general surgical service and tested for their practical consequences.

4.1.1
Definitions of SIRS, Sepsis and Septic Shock According to the Consensus Conference (Bone et al. 1992 (ACCP/CCM))

SIRS (Systemic Inflammatory Response Syndrome)

Two or more of the following conditions must be met:

Temperature of > 38 °C or < 36 °C.
Heart rate of > 90 beats/min.

Respiratory rate of > 20/min or $PaCO_2$ < 32 mm Hg.
White blood cell count of > 12 000/mm³ or < 4000/mm³.

Sepsis

Sepsis is defined as a systemic reaction of the organism to an infection with the following manifestations:

Temperature of > 38 °C or < 36 °C
Heart rate of > 90 beats/min.
Respiratory rate of > 20/min or $PaCO_2$ < 32 mm Hg.
White blood cell count of > 12 000/mm³ or < 4000/mm³.
Infection has to be proven (this means SIRS and infection).

Severe Sepsis

The patients meet the conditions of sepsis and also suffer from organ dysfunction, which is manifested by a hypoperfusion of this organ or by hypotension. The hypoperfusion of different organ systems is defined by the presence of lactic acidosis, oliguria or acute alterations in the mental state.

Septic Shock

The patients meet the criteria of severe sepsis but are hypotonic despite there being an adequate volume substitution (systolic tension < 90 mm Hg). Patients treated with vasoconstrictors are also considered to be suffering from septic shock.

4.1.2
Epidemiology of SIRS, Sepsis and Septic Shock

Within the total group of 656 patients, 335 (51.1%) patients met the criteria of SIRS. For 65 of the patients showing SIRS (corresponding to 9.9% of the total cohort), an infection could be microbiologically documented. Therefore these patients were considered to be septic according to ACCP/CCM. The remaining 270 patients (41.2% of the total group) did not show any microbiologically proven infection, and were therefore only classified as suffering from SIRS. Out of these 270 patients exclusively suffering from SIRS, 11 died. This corresponds to a SIRS mortality of 4.1%. Among the 65 septic patients, 47 (72.3% of the septic patients) developed shock. 22 (46.8%) of the patients survived. 25 patients did not survive septic shock, which corresponds to a mortality of 53.2%.

18 patients (27% of the septic patients) did not develop shock during sepsis meaning that they were neither hypotonic (systolic tension <90 mm Hg) nor permanently requiring the administration of catecholamines (during the period when they met the criteria of sepsis). Of the patients only meeting the criteria of sepsis, one patient died (mortality rate 5.6%).

Table 1.

	Normal Cohort		Pat. with SIRS only		Pat. with sepsis only		Pat. with septic shock	
	surviving	deceased	surviving	deceased	surviving	deceased	surviving	deceased
n	316	5	259	11	17	1	22	25
Women	119	3	117	6	3	1	10	8
Men	197	2	142	5	14	0	12	17
Age/years	58.7 (18–91)	67.5 (56–80)	56.5 (17–88)	57.6 (22–75)	53.5 (30–87)	84	48.6 (17–74)	61.5 (24–87)
Period of hospitalisation/days	1.6 (1–16)	2.5 (1–7)	2.7 (1–21)	3.4 (1–7)	18.7 (2–42)	6	34.2 (7–82)	17 (2–77)
Period of ventilation/days	0.15 (0–2)	0.4 (0,3–1)	0.5 (0–12,8)	1.7 (0–6)	6.5 (0–29,8)	2	23.5 (0,75–75,5)	15.4 (0,1–76,7)
Pneumonia/days	1.25 (1–2) only 8 of 316 patients had pneumonia	0	1.4 (1–3) only 22 of 259 patients had pneumonia	2.5 (2–5) 4 of 11 patients had pneumonia	1.4 (0–8) With respect to all patients	0	6.2 (0–32) With respect to all patients	3.8 (0–21) With respect to all patients
ARDS/days	0	0	2 patients during 2 days each	1 patient during one day	1,3 (0–13)	0	2.5 (0–15)	4.3 (0–40)
Hemofiltration/days	0	0	1	4 patients for 3 (1 to 6) days each 7 days	1 patient for 7 days	0	5.2 (0–49)	4.5 (0–35)
Date of death/day	/	2.5. (1–7.)	/	3.4. (1–7.)	/	6	/	17 (2–77)

The remaining 321 patients of the total group (48.9%) never met any of the required criteria of SIRS, sepsis or septic shock. Among the patients of this normal cohort, 5 died which constitutes a mortality rate of 1.5%.

4.1.3
Description of the "Normal Cohort" (see also Table 1)

The group of patients that -during the period of their stay in the intensive care unit – never met the required criteria as defined by the Consensus Conference for SIRS, sepsis or septic shock, was composed of 122 women and 199 men. 3 of the men and 2 of the women died in the intensive care unit. Therefore the total mortality rate was 1.5%.

The surviving women were on average 58.9 (19 to 91) years old, whilst the deceased women exhibited an average age of 69.5 (64 to 80) years. The group of male patients exhibited an average age of 58.5 (19 to 87) years, whilst the deceased men of the normal cohort exhibited an average age of 65.5 (56 to 75) years. An overall comparison shows that the surviving patients were, on average, 58.7 (18 to 91) years old whereas the age of the deceased patients was on average 67.5 (56 to 80) years. The average period of hospitalisation of the surviving patients was 1.6 (1 to 16) days. The deceasing patients remained in the intensive care unit for an average of 2.5 (1 to 7) days.

The surviving patients were mechanically ventilated for an average of 0.15 (0 to 2) days of their stay in the intensive care unit, this corresponds to 9.4% of their hospitalisation time. The deceasing patients were dependent on controlled ventilation for 0.4 (0.3 to 1) days, corresponding to 16% of their time in the intensive care unit.

In the group of the surviving patients, pneumonia was radiologically diagnosed in 8 patients for an average period of 1.25 (1 to 2) days. None of the deceasing patients showed any signs of pneumonia as documented by radiology. The clinical symptoms of an ARDS were not found in the surviving or the deceased patients. Neither the surviving nor the deceasing patients required hemofiltration and the date of death for the non-surviving patients was on average day 2.5 (1st to 7th day) of their hospitalisation period.

4.1.4
Analysis of Patients That Exclusively Met the Criteria of SIRS (see also Table 1)

The group of patients meeting the criteria of only SIRS according to ACCP/CCM consisted of 123 women and 147 men. Of these, 117 women survived SIRS and 6 died from it. In the male group 142 survived whereas 5 patients died of SIRS. The surviving women were on average 56.8 (17 to 88) years old, whilst the non-surviving women were 59.3 (22 to 75) years old. The surviving male patients were on average 56.1 (22 to 83) years old, differing only slightly from the average age of the deceased group (55.9 years; 24 to 74). An overall comparison revealed an average age of 56.7 (17 to 88) years for the group of surviving patients, whilst that of the non-surviving was of 57.6 (22 to 75) years. For the surviving patients, an average time of hospitalisation time of 2.7 (1 to 21) days was observed, whilst the deceased patients were the subjects of 3.4 (1 to 7) days of intensive care.

An average period of mechanical ventilation of 0.5 (0 to 12.8) days was necessary for the patients surviving SIRS. This constituted 18.5% of the hospitalisation period. The deceased patients were administered ventilation for an average of 1.7 (0 to 6) days, i.e. 50% of their intensive care period. Pneumonia was radiologically diagnosed in 22 of the patients surviving the SIRS, this being detectable for an average of 1.4 (1 to 3) days. Among the deceased patients, 4 exhibited the clinical symptoms of pneumonia with an average duration of 2.5 (2 to 5) days. Two patients surviving the SIRS showed the clinical and radiological characteristics of ARDS for one day only as did 11 of the deceased patients.

And one of the 259 surviving patients had to be hemofiltered for a period of one day whilst in the deceased patients, 4 individuals had to be hemofiltered for an average of 3 (1 to 6) days.

With respect to the definition of SIRS according to ACCP/CCM the results are as follows:

The defined parameters of temperature, pulse, leukocyte numbers, respiration and PCO_2 characteristic of SIRS were found among the surviving patients for an average period of 1.6 (1 to 7) days. This constitutes 59.3% of the hospitalisation time. The non-surviving patients displayed the symptoms of SIRS during 2.3 (1 to 5) days or 68.4% of their overall hospitalisation time. The start of SIRS was observed at day 1.4 (1 to 10) of the hospitalisation period within the surviving patient group, this did not differ greatly from the average value retained for the deceased patients (day 1.3; day 1 to 2). In general, death occurred on day 3.4 (1 to 7) of intensive care treatment.

4.1.5
Analysis of Patients That exclusively Met the Criteria for Sepsis (i.e. SIRS and Infection)

This group of patients consisted of 4 women and 14 men. Out of the 4 women, three survived the sepsis whereas one died; all male patients survived sepsis. The surviving women were on average 53.4 (38 to 64) years old, the patient who died from sepsis was 84 years old. The male patients were on average 53.6 (30 to 87) years old and the overall age of the surviving patients was 53.5 (30 to 87) years.

The duration of hospitalisation was on average 18.7 (2 to 42) days whilst the deceased patient was hospitalised for a period of six days. Surviving patients were mechanically ventilated for an average of 6.5 (0 to 29.8) days whilst the deceased patient was only ventilated for two.

In the group of surviving patients, assisted ventilation was started on day 1.4 (1st to 10th day) of the intensive care period, whereas the deceasing patient had been ventilated from the fourth day onwards. The surviving patients displayed the clinical symptoms of pneumonia for an average of 1.4 (0 to 8) days representing 7.5% of their overall hospitalisation time. In general, the pneumonia was diagnosed at day 1.4 (1st to 11th day). The deceasing patients exhibited no signs of pneumonia. The radiological characteristics of an ARDS were detected by 1.3 (0 to 13) days with the first signs occurring at day 1.1 (2nd to 12th day) of hospitalisation. Deceasing patients did not suffer from ARDS. Within the group of surviving patients, only one individual required treatment by hemofiltration this occurring at seven days. Hemofiltration was not administered to the deceasing patients.

A positive blood culture was documented as occurring four times in the group of surviving patients; the organisms detected, and their frequencies were as follows : Candida albicans 2x, Aspergillus niger and Escherichia coli 1x. It was not possible to document positive blood cultures in deceasing patients.

With respect to the definition of SIRS and sepsis according to the ACCP/CCM, the results were as follows: For an average period of 8.3 (2 to 23) days, the surviving patients met the criteria of SIRS meaning that they suffered from SIRS for 44.4% of their hospitalisation period. The female patient that did not survive sepsis fulfilled the criteria for two days of her intensive care treatment representing 33.3% of her hospitalisation period. The starting date of sepsis, defined as the time when an infection is first detectable by microbiological means and when the patient simultaneously meets the criteria of an SIRS, was found on average at day 5.5 (1st to 20th day). However the deceased patient already met these criteria at day 4 of her hospitalisation.

4.1.6
Analysis of the Patients Meeting the Criteria for Septic Shock
(see also Table 1)

This group of patients consisted of 18 women and 29 men; ten women survived their septic shock whilst 8 died. The surviving and deceased women were on average 44.4 (17 to 65) and 60.2 (42 to 81) years old, respectively. The 12 surviving men were on average aged 52.7 (27 to 74) years, and the 17 deceased men 62.2 (24 to 87) years. All in all the group of surviving patients displayed an average age of 48.6 (17 to 74) years whereas the deceased patient group were on average 61.5 (24 to 87) years old. The duration of hospitalisation was found to be 34.2 (7 to 82) and 17 (2 to 22) days for the surviving and deceasing patients, respectively.

Significant differences between the group of surviving patients and that of the deceased can be seen when the duration of assisted ventilation is expressed with respect to the total hospitalisation time. The surviving individuals were on average ventilated for a period of 23.5 (0.7 to 75.5) days which represents 68.7% of the hospitalisation period; for the deceasing individuals, an average ventilation time of 15.4 (0.1 to 76.7) days was observed, constituting 90.6% of their hospitalisation time. Controlled respiration was started at day 1.1 (1st to 4th day) for the survivors, and at day 1.9 (1st to 8th) days for non-survivors.

The clinical signs of pneumonia were detectable among the surviving patients for 6.2 (0–32) days of their intensive care stay, which represents 18.1% of their hospitalisation time. Among the deceasing patients, pneumonia was present for 3.8 (0–21) days or 22.4% of their intensive care treatment period. Whereas pneumonia was manifest at day 6.4 (3rd to 26th day) in the surviving individuals, the deceasing patients manifested pneumonia on average three days earlier, i.e. at day 3.3 (1st to 20th day).

The radiological signs of an ARDS were observed in the survivor group from day 5.5 (2nd to 40th day) onwards lasting for an average of 2.5 (0 to 15) days. With respect to their hospitalisation time, this means that they suffered from ARDS during 7.3% of their intensive care stay. In the deceased group, ARDS was diagnosed at day 6.2 (3rd to 22nd day) with an average duration of 4.3 (0 to 40) days. This represents 25.3% of their hospitalisation time and constitutes, in comparison to the surviving patients, a significant difference in the proportional duration of ARDS between the two groups analysed.

Treatment by hemofiltration was required in both groups of patients. For the surviving patients, hemofiltration was on average initiated at day 3.5 (2nd to 19th day) and continued for 5.2 (0 to 49) days, i.e. 15.2% of the hospitalisation time. In comparison, the starting date of hemofiltration of the deceasing patients was not significantly different: beginning at day 3.4 (3rd to 15th day) for an average of 4.5 (0 to 35) days representing 26.5% of this group's total hospitalisation period.

The following organisms and their incidences were detected in the positive blood culture results were obtained for 14 of the surviving patients: Candida albicans 7x, Enterobacter and Streptococcus faecalis 2x, Staphylococcus aureus and epidermidis and Pseudomonas aeruginosa 1x. In the deceased group 11 patients exhibited positive blood culture results with Candida albicans being present six times, and Streptococcus faecalis, Staphylococcus aureus, Morganella, Echinococcus alveolaris and Proteus vulgaris being detected only once.

With respect to the definitions of SIRS, sepsis and septic shock according to the ACCP/CCM we obtained the following results:

The surviving patients met the SIRS criteria for a period of 25.8 (3 to 71) days signifying that these patients can be classified as suffering from SIRS during 75.4% of their hospitalisation time, with this being attained at day 1.8 (1st to 6th day). The deceased patients exhibited SIRS for a duration of 13.8 (1 to 44) days corresponding to 81.2% of their hospitalisation period. As in the surviving patients, the start of SIRS in this group was observed at day 1.5 (1st to 5th day).

The occurrence of sepsis was found to be very similar in both groups of patients. The surviving patients were found to be septic from day 3.4 (1st to 6th day) onwards, meaning that an infection was microbiologically detectable at that date. In the deceased patients, an infection was detected at day 3.7 (1st to 6th day).

Septic shock was symptomatically detected in the surviving patients at day 5.4 (1st to 22nd day) for an average duration of 10.3 (1 to 30) days, representing 31.1% of their hospitalisation time. The deceased patients exhibited the initial signs of septic shock at day 5 (1st to 23rd day), for an average of 8.1 (1 to 19) days. In comparison to the surviving patients this latter value should be analysed as a proportion of the total hospitalisation time. In fact, the deceasing patients suffered from septic shock during 47.6% of their ICU time, this being significantly longer than in the surviving individuals. The patients not surviving the septic shock died, on average, on day 17 (2nd to 77th day) of their ICU stay.

4.1.7
Critical Analysis of Different Definitions of Sepsis

The endeavour of coherently defining a patient suffering from sepsis is reflected by the wealth of literature that can be found on the definition of sepsis and septic shock. In 1991 R.C. Bone, who often criticised different definitions of sepsis (Bone 1991), initiated an attempt to create common definitions of sepsis. By doing so, he was aiming to make earlier diagnosis possible, to point out risk factors that increase the probability of septic pathogenesis and that need to be observed during administration of the patient, and finally to render therapeutic approaches comparable (Bone 1994). The commonly used expression of septicaemia that describes a systemic pathogenesis of micro-organisms growing in the blood, should no longer be used as it is being used to represent different terms and the inconsistency of its use only leads to confusion. In contrast, Sprung (Sprung 1991) uses the term septicaemia as an important differentiating trait: This term describes a bacteraemia whereas he describes the consequent reaction of the organism as sepsis.

R.C. Bone defines sepsis by physiologically measurable parameters (Bone 1991): tachypnea (with respiration rate of >20/min), tachycardia (heart rate of >90 beats/min), hypo- or hyperthermia (temperature of $<35.5°C$ or $>38°C$). Accordingly, these clinical alterations are the proof of sepsis. Furthermore, Bone uses the term septic syndrome, with which he associates the term sepsis, but in addition takes into account changes in organ perfusion. Alertness of the patient diminishes dramatically, the PaO_2/FiO_2 ratio drops below 280, lactic acidosis increases and an oliguria (0.5 ml/kg/KG/h) can be observed. Furthermore Bone defines septic shock as a septic syndrome with an accompanying hypotension (systolic tension of <90 mm Hg) that can be cured by the adequate administration of isotonic crystalloids or catecholamines. Finally Bone uses the term of refractory septic shock. In this state the patient is hypotonic for more than one hour and the hypotony cannot be overcome by adequate treatment.

The terminology introduced by R. C. Bone has been appreciated as an attempt to create general definitions (Sibbald et al. 1991); however critics consider them to be imprecise. The use of these definitions is unable to discount for the lack of standardisation in the judgement of septic patients. A terminology of sepsis has to take into account that sepsis and infection can constitute not only a reaction to the invasive micro-organism but also a corporal response to the infection.

In the definitions of sepsis, the complex interplay between the invasion of the micro-organism and the reaction of the host is not sufficiently taken into consideration. Thus the clinical proof of an infection is completely lacking from Bone's definitions. For instance, the secretion of factors such as tumour necrosis factor can occur in the absence of an infection and lead to reactions in the organism, which resemble that of an infection leading to the clinical signs of sepsis.

To solve these problems the Consensus Conference was organised in 1991. Its aims were not only to define sepsis and septic shock in a general and reliable way but also to give practical advice as to how patients can unequivocally be recognised as being septic. This terminology should be used clinically as well as in newly appearing studies so that comparable contingencies of patients would arise. During this conference a new term, the SIRS, was created. This term is meant to describe the reaction of the body by showing the same clinical symptoms as sepsis, which can be seen in case of certain infections (tachycardia, fever or hyperventilation). Only in case of a microbiologically detectable infection the patient can be considered to be septic. This clearly constitutes a difference to R. C. Bone's definitions of the septic syndrome, which, even when an infection is only suspected, considers the patient to be septic.

A study comprising 210 surgical patients addressed the question as to whether a documented infection was pertinent for the diagnosis and the prognosis of sepsis (Marshall and Sweeney, 1990). The results showed that infection constitutes a microbiological phenomenon, that the body reacts to this invasion of microorganisms and that any further outcome was influenced not only by the gravity of this reaction but also by the general constitution of the patient (Parillo 1993). However, the detection of infection was not linked to the further pathogenesis of sepsis (Marshall and Sweeney, 1990). This would be in accordance with Bone's proposition but not with that of the Consensus Conference, which demanded a documented infection as an initial criterion for sepsis. This notion of an absolute requirement of a documented infection is criticised by Vincent (Vincent 1997). He realised the difficulties of providing this proof for traumatised patients that show the signs of sepsis despite the lack of an obvious infectious focus. With respect to this, the Consensus Conference attempted to attribute the term SIRS to this non-infectious cause of sepsis. It should be pointed out here that SIRS (i.e. without documented infection) and sepsis (i.e. with documented infection) could obviously exhibit identical clinical symptoms (Schein et al. 1997).

The participants of the Consensus Conference further defined the term of severe sepsis. During this severe form of sepsis, the patients display the signs of organ hypoperfusion. Again, we can see a great deal of similarity with the term of septic syndrome by R. C. Bone (Bone 1991). The additional problems such as an alteration in mental function are considered to be an early sign of the deterioration in the septic pathology, but these can only be poorly verified with intubated and ventilated patients . Other abnormalities such as lactic acidosis and oliguria can more easily give an indication of deterioration. The definition of septic shock implies sepsis and additionally a clear hypotension (systolic tension < 90 mm Hg): Patients treated with vasoactive drugs do not show any signs of hypotension but can still be considered to be suffering from septic shock.

As outlined above, the definitions of the Consensus Conference are not generally accepted, but it has been requested to work with this new terminology in order to define its practicability in clinical life (Sibbald et al. 1995).

4.1.8
Comparison of Distinct Studies Having Applied the Definitions of the Consensus Conference (Table 2)

When comparing distinct studies, we conclude that the definitions of the Consensus Conference have lead to different results. In Italy (Salvo et al. 1995) and

Table 2.

	Frankfurt	Italy (Salvo et al. 1995)	USA/Switzerland Study I (Rangel-Frausto et al. 1995)	USA/Switzerland Study II (Pittet et al. 1995)	France (Bruin-Buisson et al. 1995)
Contingency of patients of the analysed intensive care unit	Patients of general surgery	Patients of internal medicine and surgery	Patients of internal medicine and surgery	Surgical patients	Patients of internal medicine and surgery
Total group	656	1100	3708	170	11740
SIRS	335	573	2527	158	Not Determined
Patient(s)	51.1% of total group	52% of total group	68.1% of total group	93% of total group	Not Determined
Sepsis	65	50	649	83	
Patient(s)	10% of total group	4.5% of total group	17.5% of total group	49% of total group	
Severe Sepsis	[a]	23	467	28	742
Patient(s)		2.1% of total group	12.6% of total group	16.5% of total group	6.3% of total group
Septic Shock	47	33	110	12	528
Patient(s)	7% of total group	3% of total group	3% of total group	7% of total group	4.5% of total group
Source of Infection Microbiologically Documented?	yes	yes	yes [b]	Infection not documented for all cases [c]	yes

[a] Patients included in the "septic shock" group.

[b] This study analysed patients with a documented infection as well as those with a suspected infection (who were therefore treated with antibiotics). Only patients with a documented infection are shown in this table.

[c] The suspicion of (patient was treated with antibiotics for more than 72 h) as well as a verified source of infection was considered an infection.

Frankfurt the clinical state of SIRS was seen at similar rates for patients in the intensive care unit. In both studies, more than 50% of all patients exhibited the symptoms of SIRS. We would like to point out clearly that the two studies did not deal with comparable, homogenous cohorts of patients. Our study deals exclusively with surgical patients whereas the Italian study is based on a mixed group of patients. The Italian study critically states that certain factors of SIRS are easily observable in patients admitted for internal medical services. Many patients suffering from cardiac insufficiencies are tachycardic in the absence of an infectious cause. Moreover, tachycardia caused by a non-infectious pathogenesis is a frequent diagnosis for post-surgical patients suffering from anxiety, stress or slight hypovolemia.

The two other studies from the USA and Switzerland, describe significantly higher incidences of SIRS. In study I, dealing with a mixed group of patients (Rangel-Frausto et al. 1995), frequencies are somewhat lower (68%) as in study II, which exclusively takes into account surgical patients (Pittet et al. 1995). In the latter study, nearly all patients met the criteria of an SIRS. Therefore the authors do not consider the term SIRS to be of significance for prognosis. This means that the term SIRS is sensitive, but it is not specific enough. In comparison to the Frankfurt group of patients that met the SIRS criteria we are led to similar conclusions: sensitivity was 88% and specificity 51% with respect to the criteria of survival or death.

With respect to the number of patients suffering from sepsis, similar differences can be observed. The frequencies of sepsis among patients vary from 4.5% (Italy) to 49% (USA/Switzerland). In search of the causes for these discrepancies, one is forced to realise that the criteria defining sepsis were applied in a quite different manner. In our study, a patient was only considered to be septic when a microorganism (infection) was successfully documented. The same categorisation of septic patients was also used in Italy. In comparison to the 10% of patients that were assigned as being septic in Frankfurt, less were found in Italy (4.5%). Studies I and II however, show a different use of the term "infection". In Study I, a division is made between culture-positive sepsis (documented infection) and culture-negative sepsis (suspected infection). Study II talks about a "suspected infection" when the patient had been administered an antibiotic treatment for more than 72 hours even if no source of infection was found. In this study, sepsis is diagnosed as such when SIRS is "thought to be caused" by an infection. This does not meet the definition of the Consensus Conference and has therefore been criticised by others (Sibbald et al. 1995). If one only takes into consideration the patients in study II that truly meet the criteria of sepsis (n = 33), this corresponds to an incidence of 19.4%. This value corresponds well with results from other studies.

The incidences of septic shock are similar in all studies ranging between 3 to 7%. From this it can be concluded that the diagnosis of "septic shock" as defined by the Consensus Conference leads to a similar contingency of patients. This is particularly so when results from different studies are compared and it becomes evident that the creation of common groups of patients is necessary to enable pertinent comparison of terms.

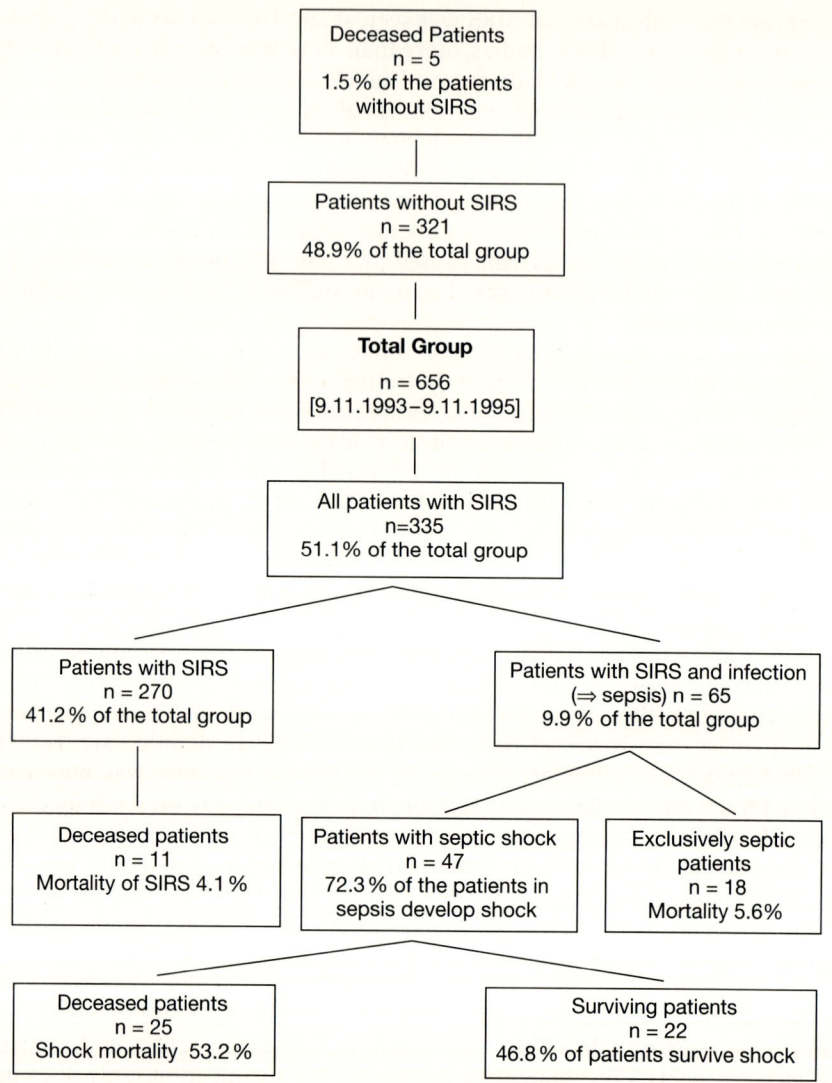

Fig. 1.

A French multi-centre study (Bruin-Buisson et al. 1995) which also applied the terminology of the Consensus Conference came up with the following results:

Out of 11740 patients under observation, 1052 showed the clinical symptoms of severe sepsis, of these the infection could also be microbiologically documented in 742 patients (6.3%).

This analysis included patients admitted to internal medical (64%), surgical (with planned and emergency interventions) or trauma services (36%).

Of the 742 patients with a documented infection, only 528 patients (4.5% of the total cohort) were diagnosed as suffering from septic shock. No significant difference was observed between patients with a documented infection and those with a suspected infection. Both groups of patients displayed similar symptoms of "severe sepsis", such as metabolic acidosis and oliguria. Differences were only visible for patients with suspected sepsis (so-called culture-negative sepsis) who showed a higher incidence of hypotension than those with a documented infection (sepsis).

This study (Bruin-Buisson et al. 1995) was aiming to clarify whether, in terms of clinical parameters, risk factors or prognosis, a distinction can be made between patients with a verified or suspected infection. The study could not come up with significant differences and therefore, as already discussed elsewhere (Rangel-Frausto et al. 1995) the terms of SIRS and sepsis were considered to be difficult to separate. For this reason, the authors (Bruin-Buisson et al. 1995) suggest that, besides the definitions and terminology of the Consensus Conference, other scoring systems such as APACHE III or SAPS II should be considered in order to establish a prognosis.

In summary, we conclude that the terms of SIRS and sepsis as defined by the Consensus Conference have little impact on the clinical treatment of our patients. This is also reflected in the very different frequencies reported by other studies. However, the term septic shock, defines a group of high-risk patients, which are worthwhile further characterising.

4.2
Description of Sequential Organ Failure in Critically Ill Abdominal Surgical Patients

In 1994 the "Working Group on Sepsis-Related Problems of the European Society of Intensive Care Medicine" developed a scoring system at a Consensus Conference in Paris. The proposed scoring system aimed on the one hand to improve the current understanding of the progression of organ dysfunction and the failure of an organ system and on the other hand to describe the impact of a given therapy on the organ dysfunction or failure (Vincent et al. 1996). This score was intended to be based on parameters, which are as objective and easily determinable so that the score would be largely free of errors of judgement and also routinely applicable.

This score was called the "sepsis-related organ failure assessment (SOFA) score". First of all, this score was developed to describe the damage to the different organ systems. However, given that damage of organs and mortality are related it was questioned as to whether this score could also be used to predict patient survival. In this study we have addressed the question as to whether the SOFA-score can be used to make a prediction of mortality in patients in an intensive care unit. For comprehension, the results were compared to those achieved using the APACHE II and the MOD-scoring systems (Marshall et al. 1995). In particular, we further established a "receiving operating characteristic"-curve

Table 3. Definitions of the SOFA-score

SOFA-Score	1	2	3	4
Respiratory Score (PaO$_2$/FiO$_2$ in mmHg)	<400	<300	<200 with mechanical ventilation	<100 with mechanical ventilation
Coagulation Score (thrombocytes $\times 10^3$/mm^3)	<150	<100	<50	<20
Hepatic Score (bilirubin mg/dl (µmol/l))	1.2–1.9 (20–32)	2.0–5.9 (33–101)	6.0–11.9 (102–204)	>12.0 (>204)
Circulatory Score Hypotension (doses in µg/kg $\times$ min)	MAP <70 mm Hg	Administration of dopamine ≤5 or dobutamine	Administration of >5 dopamine or ≤0.1 catecholamine	Administration of >15 dopamine or <0.1 catecholamine
CNS-Score (Glasgow-Coma-Score)	13–14	10–12	6–9	<6
Renal Score (creatinine mg/dl (µmol/l) or diuresis ml/day)	1.2–1.9 (110–170)	2.0–3.4 (171–299)	3.5–4.9 (300–440) (200–500)	>5.0 (>440) (<200)

(ROC-curve) (Hanley and McNeil, 1982) from these scores in order to assess their significance.

SOFA-Score (Vincent et al. 1996)
A slightly modified SOFA-score was determined for every patient and day of hospitalisation, this was because the determination of the CNS-score proved to be unreliable as it could not be unambiguously stated as to whether a patient had attained the respective Glasgow-Coma-Scale values because of the necessary sedation or due to a defect of the CNS; this difficulty has also been recorded by Bein et al. (1995) and Bastos et al. (1993). For this reason the CNS-score was not taken into consideration for the determination of the SOFA-score.

The SOFA-score was determined according to the definition shown in Table 3. The highest respective day value is given.

APACHE II (Knaus et al. 1985)
According to the scoring system developed by Knaus et al. the APACHE II score was determined on the first day of intensive care, SIRS, sepsis and of septic shock, respectively.

MOD-Score (Marshall et al. 1995)
The MOD-score was calculated from Table 4. Values were determined on the first day of hospitalisation, SIRS, sepsis and of septic shock, respectively.

ROC Analysis
The ROC analysis has become a standard in the comparative assessment of score systems. The area value under the curve gives an indication of the quality and reliability of a scoring system with respect to a given question.

Table 4. Definitions of the MOD-score

Organ System	Score 0	Score 1	Score 2	Score 3	Score 4
Respiratory System (PO_2/FiO_2)	>300	226–300	151–225	76–150	≤75
Renal System (serum creatinine in µmol/l)	≤100	101–200	201–350	351–500	>500
Hepatic system (serum bilirubin in µmol/l)	≤20	21–60	61–120	121–240	>240
Cardio-vascular system (PAR= beats × ZVD/ mean. art. pressure	≤10.0	10.1–15.0	15.1–20.0	20.1–30.0	>30.0
Coagulation (thrombocytes ($10^3 \cdot ml^{-1}$)	>120	81–120	51–80	21–50	≤20
Neurology/CNS (Glasgow Coma Score)	15	13–14	10–12	7–9	≤6

To calculate the ROC curve, the respective score has to be determined for each case. In addition, a null hypothesis is established with respect to the question to be analysed.

The following is an example for such a calculation and is given for the prediction of the survival of patients.

1. Score calculation for all patients on the first day of their hospitalisation.
2. Fixing a threshold value (cut-off-point), on reaching or exceeding this score-value X, the patient will die.
3. Calculating the sensitivity and specificity for all possible values (X) of the score. For instance, in case of the APACIIE II score, it can vary from 0 to 70.
4. The values of the specificity are converted into the form of a "1-specificity".
5. Pairs of values for the sensitivity and the "1-specificity" are grouped into a table.
6. Subsequently a curve is established with the values of the 1-specificity and of the sensitivity on the x- and y-axis, respectively.

By plotting the curves and calculating the area under the curve, the quality of each scoring system can be evaluated with respect to the given question. A good scoring system is characterised by area values greater than 0.8. A value of 0.5 represents the probability of being able to predict the result by tossing a coin. The system achieving the highest area value is considered to be most suitable to answer any given question. These curves were calculated using the MOD, APACHE II and SOFA score on the first day of hospitalisation, for SIRS, sepsis and septic shock, respectively.

Table 5. Example of the determination of the SOFA-score for a patient. Values of pertinent parameters on the respective days of hospitalisation:

	Day 1	Day 2	Day 3	Day 4
PaO$_2$ (mmHg)	89	80	75	50
FiO$_2$ (%)	40	40	60	80
Thrombocytes ($\times 10^3$/mm^3)	120	80	90	110
Bilirubin (mg/dl)	4.8	6.8	3.5	1.9
Mean arterial tension (mmHg)	89	82	76	34
Dopamine (µg/kg KG × min)	0	1.2	1.2	6
Dobutamine (µg/kg KG × min)	0	0	0	2
Catecholamine (µg/kg KG × min)	0	0	0.4	1
Glasgow-Coma-Scale	11	11	9	7
Creatinine (mg/dl)	0.9	1.5	2.2	4.5
Diuresis (ml/d)	1600	1000	300	120

From this and according to the definitions given in tables 1 and 2, the following scores result for the respective days of hospitalisation:

	Day 1	Day 2	Day 3	Day 4
Respiratory Score	22	2	3	4
Coagulation-Score	1	2	2	1
Hepatic Score	2	3	2	1
Circulation-Score	0	2	4	4
CNS-Score	2	2	3	3
Renal Score	0	1	3	4
Daily Score	7	12	17	17

During the period of analysis the patient has a mean score of:
Respiration: 2.75
Coagulation: 1.5
Hepatic: 2
Circulatory: 2.5
CNS: 2.5
Renal: 2
Total: 13.25

Score Progression

To calculate and show score progression, mean score values for each patient and the day of hospitalisation were determined (see an example of the determination of the SOFA-score for a patient in table 5). In the same way, the summed scores of each day were also calculated. The data thus determined were then represented graphically. Mortality was calculated for each of the score groups. To be able do this, patients were divided into groups with respect to their mean scores

Table 6. Classification of the patients into the different categories of sepsis.

Without SIRS	383 Patients (43.8%)
With SIRS	368 Patients (42.1%)
With Sepsis	53 Patients (6.1%)
With Septic Shock	70 Patients (8.0%)

during the period of hospitalisation. Then the mortality within each group was compared.

We analysed data from 874 patients with a mean age of 58.1 (from 15 to 91) years. No significant differences in age were seen for patients of differing sex or belonging to different categories of sepsis. Of the 874 patients, 526 (60.2%) were male and 348 (39.8%) female. In total, 72 patients (8.2%) died whilst being treated in the intensive care unit; of these, 32 were female (44,4%) and 40 male (55,6%). Time of hospitalisation was on average 5.6 (1 to 109) days. The mean period of hospitalisation was 4.8 (1 to 109) days for the surviving, and 15.2 (1 to 78) days for the deceased patients. Patients were classed into the different categories of sepsis as shown in Table 5. As shown in this listing 56.2% met the criteria of a SIRS and 25.1% of these developed sepsis. For 56.9% of the septic patients, the determined parameters corresponded to septic shock.

The mortality of patients in each category of sepsis is shown in Table 6. The admission scores of patients that died during intensive care were not found to differ significantly from those of the surviving patients. The progression of the SOFA and the mean scores during the period of hospitalisation is shown in Fig. 2 and does not reveal any significant differences. With respect to mortality, a significant difference ($p < 0.001$) was seen between patients with a SOFA-score of less than 3 and those with a score of 3 (Fig. 3). The difference between the different groups and the group "score = 3" was also significant ($p < 0.001$): $r = 0.445$, $p = 0.01$ (calculated according to Pearson). The analysis of the MOD-, APACHE II- and SOFA-scores led to the generation of the ROC curves shown in Figures 4 to 7. The area under the curves was found to vary between 0.70–0.78.

Vincent et al., who created the SOFA score, reported (Vincent et al. 1998) that the SOFA-score is not only suitable for septic patients but also for all patients in an intensive care unit, namely to evaluate the state of different organ systems. That is why they suggested re-naming this score the "Sequential Organ Failure Assessment Score". Our study, with the basic data not differing much from other studies of sepsis (Pittet et al. 1995; Bruin-Buisson et al. 1995), also corroborates the results of Vincent et al. (1998). The SOFA score is a simple system that can be easily applied in the daily life of an intensive care unit. It lacks the complicated calculations that are necessary in most other scoring systems. From our results it was evident that the scores could also be consulted to evaluate the organ function of patients not suffering from sepsis. Therefore, and according to Ohmann and Groß-Weege (Ohmann and Groß-Weege, 1992), the SOFA score can be considered to be a "score covering different pathologies". Furthermore our results suggested a significant relationship between a high mean SOFA score and mortality (Fig. 2). An increase in the mean score by a factor of two to three resulted

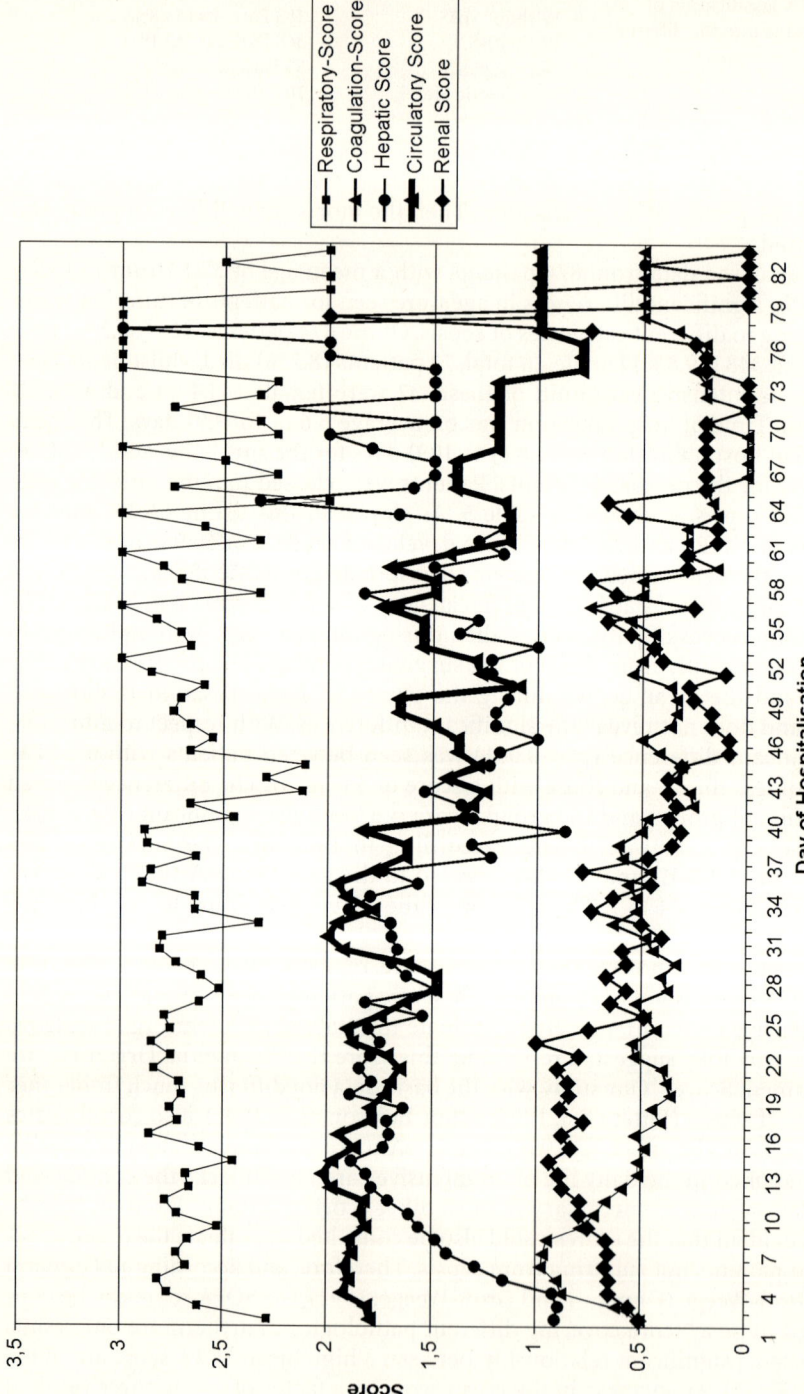

Fig. 2. Score progression as a function of hospitalisation time

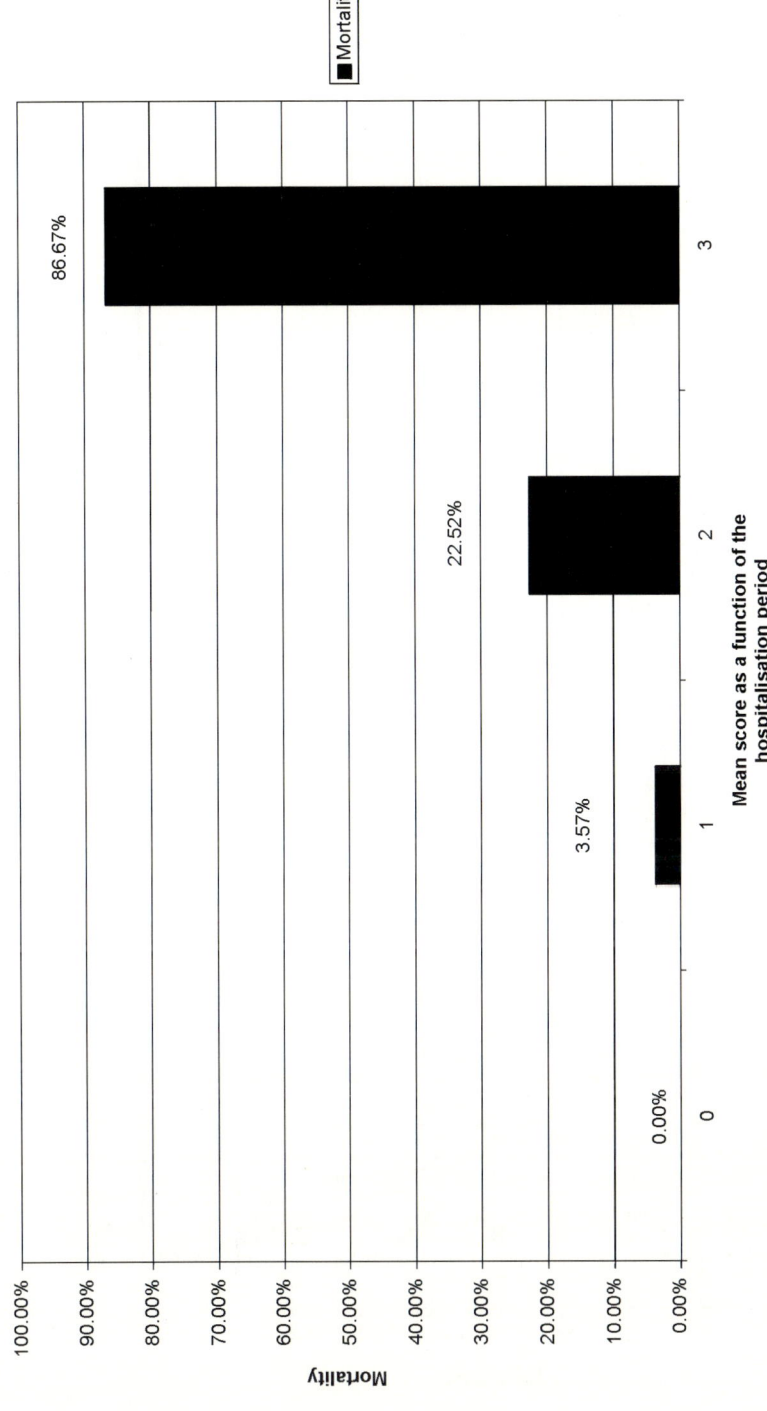

Fig. 3. Mortality depending on the SOFA-mean-score as a function of hospitalisation time

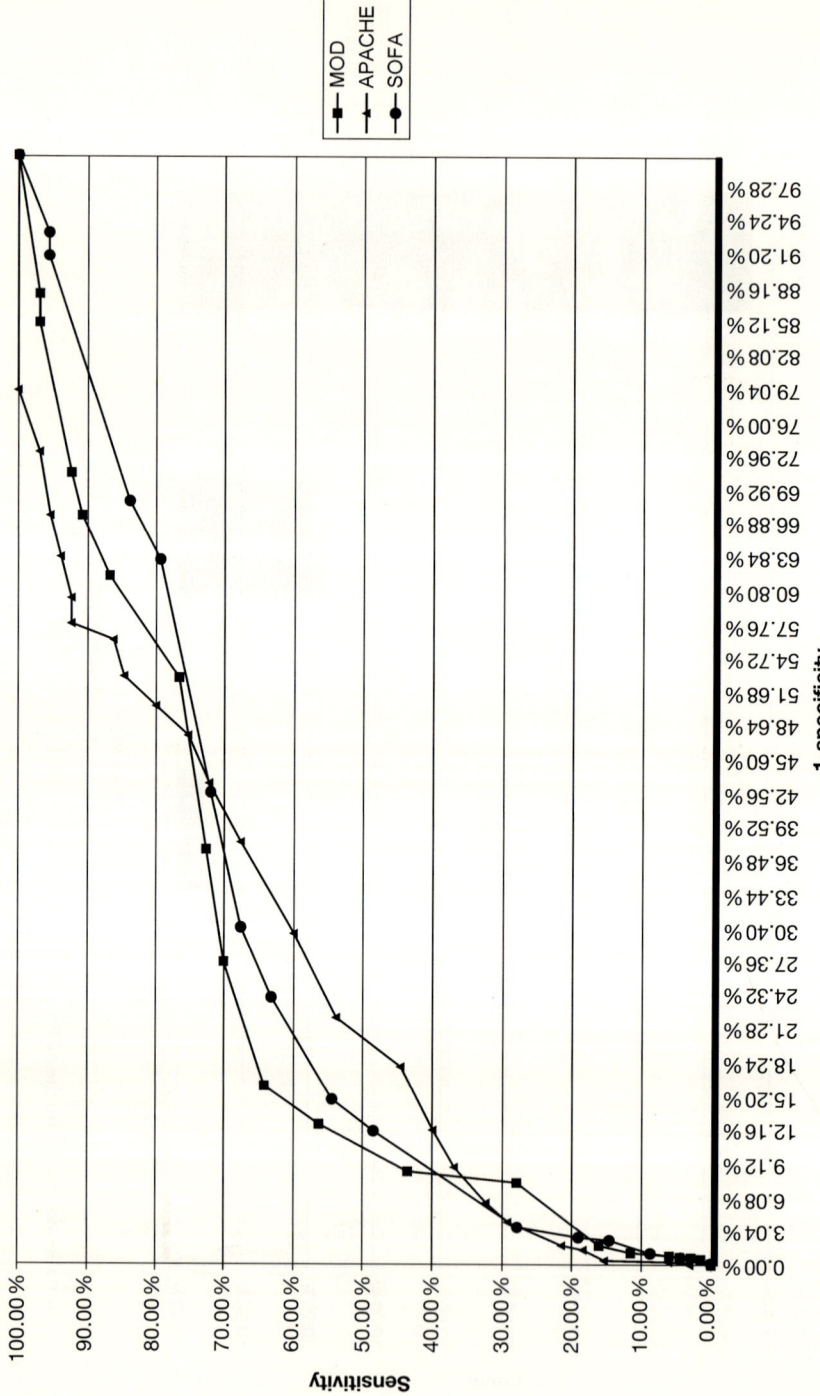

Fig. 4. ROC analysis on the first day of hospitalisation; Area under curve APACHE II: 0.74; MOD: 0.76; SOFA: 0.72

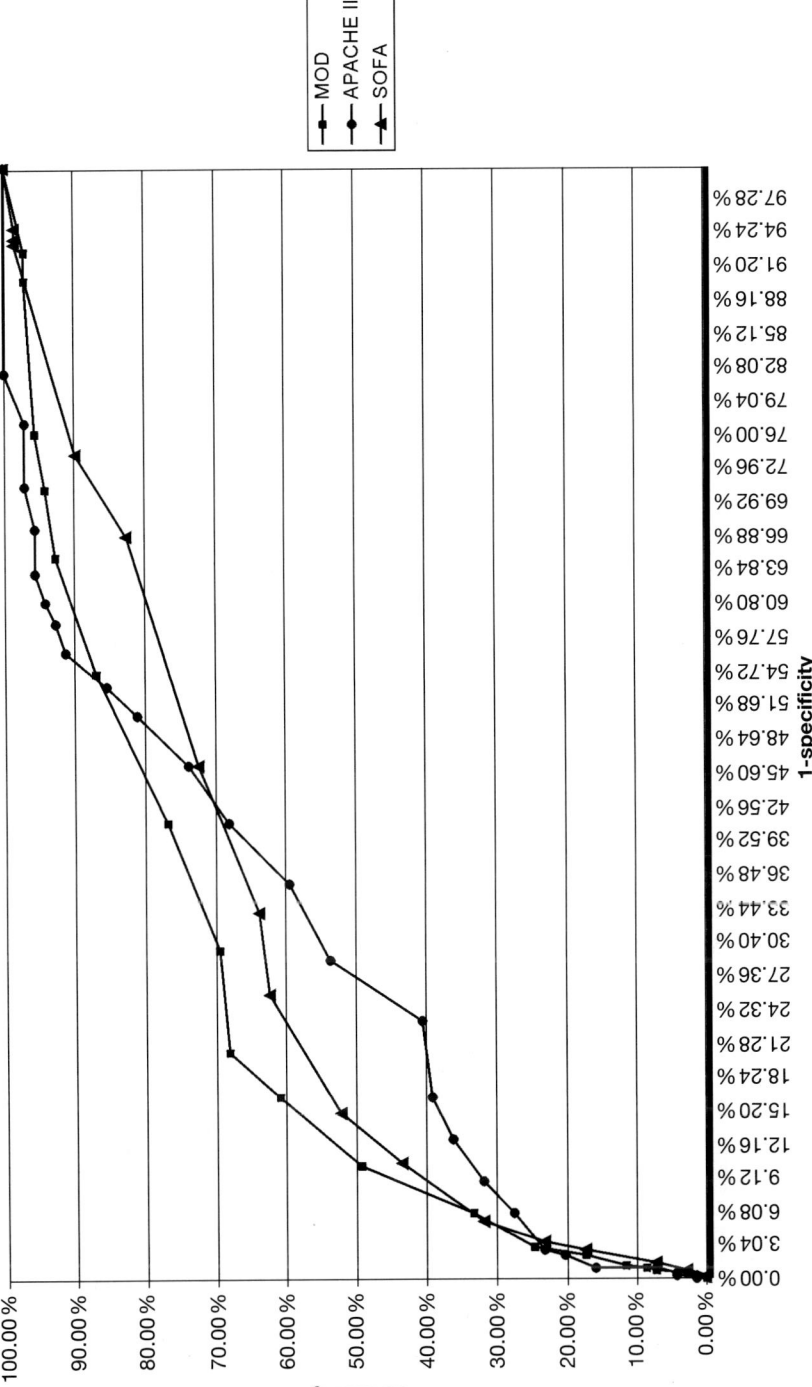

Fig. 5. ROC analysis on the first day of SIRS; Area under curve APACHE II: 0.72; MOD: 0.78; SOFA: 0.72

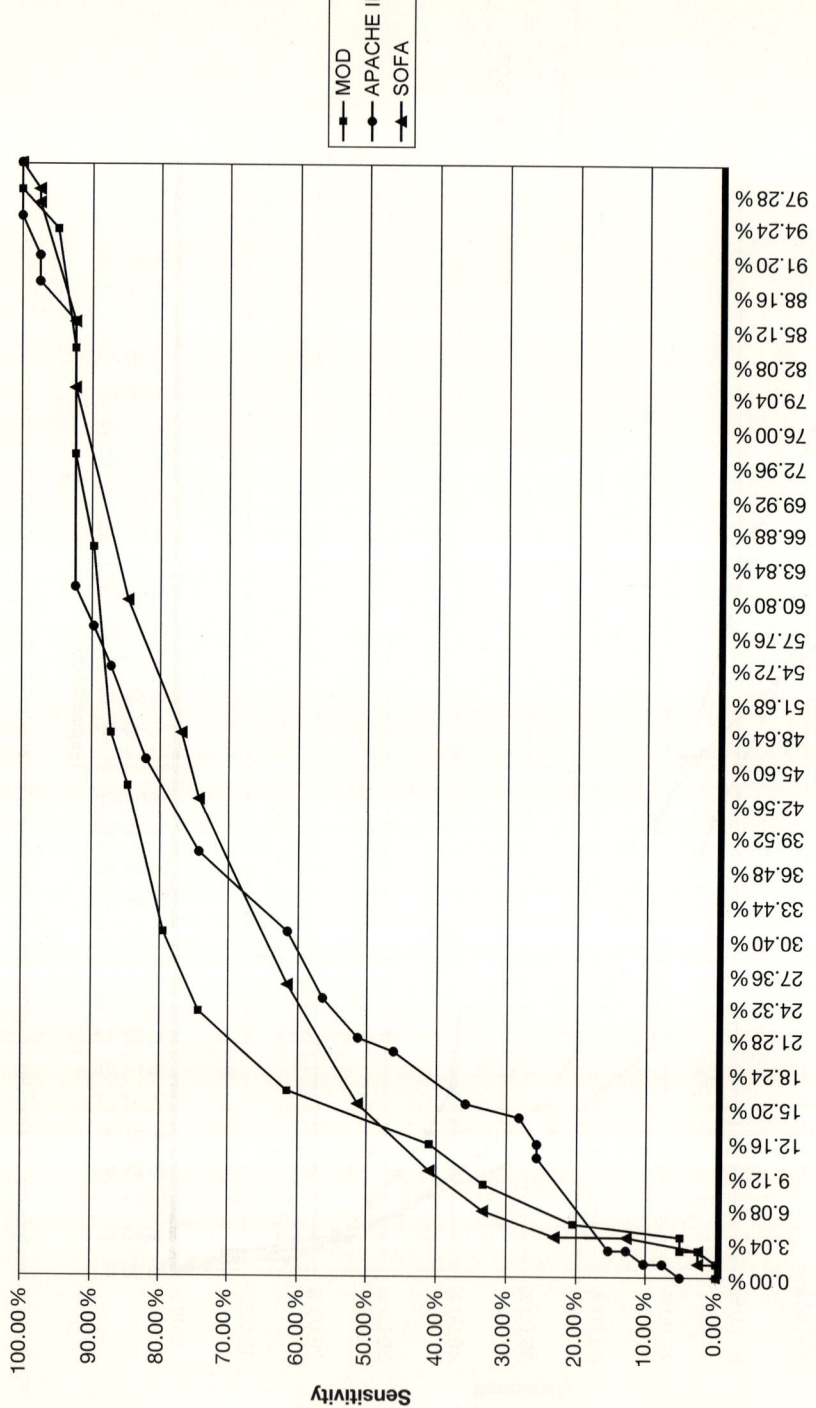

Fig. 6. ROC analysis on the first day of sepsis; Area under curve APACHE II: 0.72; MOD: 0.77; SOFA: 0.72

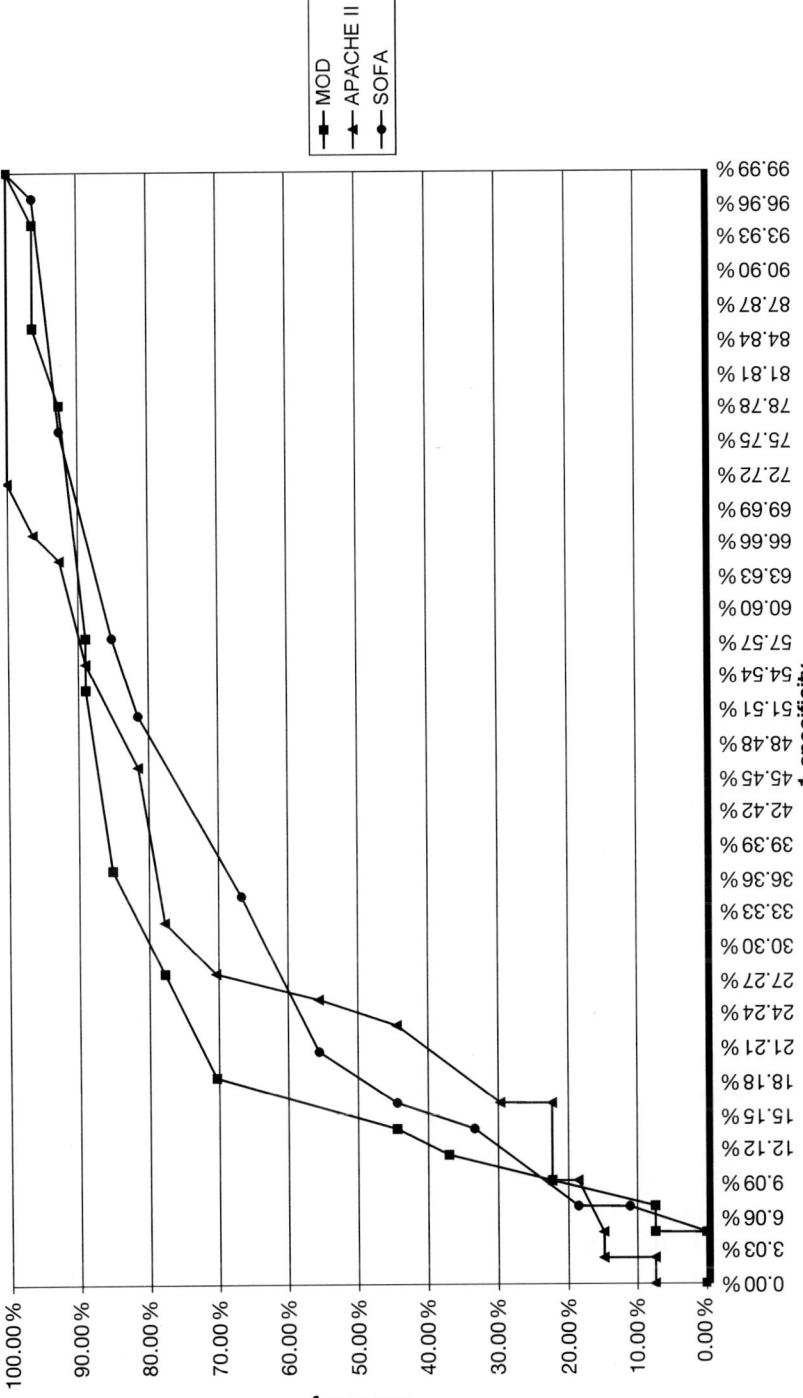

Fig. 7. ROC analysis on the first day of septic shock; Area under curve APACHE II: 0.74; MOD: 0.77; SOFA: 0.70

Table 7. Mortality within the different categories of sepsis; the admission scores are the mean scores of patients when admitted to the intensive care unit; in parenthesis the values for the survived and deceased patients

Category of sepsis	Total group of patients [n]	Deceased (n)	Mortality (%)	Admission score APACHE II (× mean)	Admission score SOFA (× mean)	Admission score MOD (× mean)
Without SIRS	383	3	0.8	11.8 (14/11.8)	4.8 (3.0/4.8)	4.5 (2.0/4.5)
With SIRS	368	30	8.2	15.2 (20.5/14.8)	5.7 (8.2/5.4)	6.1 (9.6/5.8)
With Sepsis	53	12	22.6	15.8 (20.4/14.4)	6.9 (8.0/6.5)	7.4 (9.3/6.8)
With Septic Shock	70	27	38.5	17.5 (19.6/16.3)	7.7 (9.0/6.9)	8.7 (10.1/7.8)

in a seven times higher risk of mortality. This is in accordance with the results of Vincent et al. (1998).

A comparison by ROC analysis of the SOFA score with the APACHE II and MOD scores revealed an equivalence of all these scores in predicting mortality. Only the MOD score achieved values, which were slightly better, although not significantly so. Interestingly, none of the three scores met the quality required for a good score with area values under the curve of more than 0.8 (see ROC analysis). It is, however, not our intention to interpret this observation that to all the "old, bad" scores a "new and equally bad" score has been added. Despite all their limitations, score systems do substantially contribute to describing the intensive care progression of critically ill patients. The results of the analyses of Vincent et al. as well as those undertaken on our cohort and especially their comparison with the APACHE II and MOD scores demonstrate that, in every way, the meaningfulness of the SOFA score is equal to that of other scores (APACHE II and MOD). The slight restrictions in comparison to the MOD score are, in our opinion, outweighed by the simple applicability. This is a factor already claimed for by Ohmann in 1992 (Ohmann and Groß-Weege, 1992), where all complicated calculations are discarded. However, the practical applicability of scoring systems in a daily routine was not the central point of the present study. This aspect has to be verified, which means that it should be evaluated which score best meets the demands of practical application.

These scores do not allow definite statements on individual patients, only on groups of patients (i.e. in comparative studies of groups of patients or of quality management). Therefore it remains to be tested if other data tools such as neuronal networks turn out to be useful in achieving prognosis and therapy on an individual basis.

4.3
Peritonitis

4.3.1
Definition and Causes

The term peritonitis describes an infection of the abdominal cavity, which when left untreated, rapidly leads to multi-organ dysfunction. Its pathogenesis is characterised by the paraphrased or diffuse liberation of bacteria from the intraperitoneal organs (spontaneous or iatrogenic perforation). Some rare forms of peritonitis do not emanate from the peritoneal cavity or are not primarily due to bacterial or fungal infection. They are termed primary peritonitis as opposed to the much more frequently observed secondary peritonitis.

Forms of Peritonitis and Their Causes

Primary   Spontaneous bacterial peritonitis in the case of liver cirrhosis.

Secondary   Appendicitis.
              Cholecystitis.
              Perforation of the stomach, the small or large intestine (ulcer, Crohn's disease, colitis ulcerosa, diverticulitis).
              Intestinal ischemia.
              Post-surgical peritonitis (suture failure).

4.3.2
Diagnosis

The diagnosis of peritonitis is linked to the term of an acute abdomen which is typically sudden or convulsive, very painful and often critical in disease of the abdomen. The main symptoms of the acute abdomen are as follows: spontaneous or palpation-induced pain, cramping of the abdominal wall, ileus and shock.

Many extra-abdominal diseases can cause acute abdominal pain and a differential diagnosis should by considered in the case of an acute abdomen; these include: thoracic (myocardial infarction, pericarditis, pleuritis, pulmonary embolism), neurological (herpes zoster, meningitis) and urological (nephrolithiasis) diagnoses. Certain metabolic diseases (porphyria, diabetes), intoxications and retro-peritoneal pathogeneses (psoas abscess) can also feign an acute abdomen.

Diagnosis should be corroborated by the patient's history, a physical examination, emergency lab studies, electrocardiograms, thoracic and abdominal radiographs, diuresis, sonography, computer tomography (especially for immune-compromised and elderly patients) and possibly by laparoscopy to enlarge the diagnostic spectrum.

4.3.3
Therapy

4.3.3.1
Surgical Infection Control

The strategy for treating secondary peritonitis is controlling the source of infection. This means in cases like appendicites and cholecystitis performing an appendectomy and cholecystectomy. Perforation of the stomach or duodenum will be managed by excision and suturing, alternatively by resection.

Localised abdominal infection in contrast to generalised peritonitis not necessarily needs to be treated surgically. The development of effective interventional techniques meanwhile has led to a high success rate in treating e.g. postoperative abscess formations.

Right-Sided Emergencies of the Colon

Right-sided colonic ischemia and necrosis may best be treated by right hemicolectomy or extended right hemicolectomy with primary anastomosis. In case ischemic colitis with perforation is associated with generalized peritonitis, we perform a resection with terminal ileostomy and distal colonic mucocutaneous fistula.

Left-Sided Emergencies of the Colon

Two principal alternatives are available: (1) resection of diseased intestine with delayed anastomosis (Hartmann procedure) and (2) resection with primary anastomosis. Resection of rectosigmoid carcinoma with intraperitoneal closure of the rectal stump and a terminal left iliac fossa colostomy was first described in 1921 by Hartmann (Hartmann 1921). While largely abandoned as an elective operation, many surgeons regard it as the procedure of choice for left-sided colonic emergencies. The diseased portion of intestine is removed, and hazards of an anastomosis with large intestine in the presence of peritonitis are avoided. The extent of resection should be guided by the distribution of disease as seen on the appearance of the serosal surface of the colon at the time of operation. As in all resections for colonic ischemia, the specimen must be opened the time of operation to ensure normal mucosa at the margins. If ischemic colitis involves the rectum, a mucotaneous fistula of the distal stump or a Hartmann procedure with a terminal colostomy should be performed. The mucous fistula can be fashioned within diseased bowel, providing the chance to heal with subsequent restoration of bowel continuity (Brandt and Boley 1992). It is important to be aware in this context of the frequent association of colonic ischemia with other lesions of the large bowel, such as carcinoma, diverticulitis, volvulus or fecal impaction (Boley et al. 1992). In instances where colonic ischemia occurs following surgery for abdominal aortic aneurysms, a primary anastomosis is contraindicated because of the potential danger of an intestinal leak and contamination of the aortic prothesis (Betzler 1998). The management of the rare fulminating type of colon ischemia involving all or most of the colon and rectum requires colectomy with terminal ileostomy. In some patients a second-stage proctectomy has been necessary. Mortality and morbidity rates for reversal of the Hartmann procedure are mainly known from surgery for cancer and diverticulosis, and are as follows (data are means and range; stated as percentages): deaths 4% (0–11); leak 10% (0–30); stenosis 1.5% (0–9) (Doberneck 1991). Furthermore, a large proportion of patients, in some series up to 100%, may never proceed to reversal, mainly for medical reasons. As a consequence, they are left with a permanent end colostomy. Moreover, it is recognized that stomas being applied during the course of emergency surgical treatment are frequently improperly sited and associated with a high incidence of complications. Since stoma construction and subsequent closure are associated with a considerable mortality and morbidity (Khoury et al. 1996), the concept of resection with primary anastomosis has therefore come into focus. It is generally accepted that one of the most important barriers to successful anastomotic healing is the unprepared proximal colon (Smith et al. 1983; O'Higging 1989; Irvin and Goligher 1970). Similarly, surgeons believe that peritonitis further increases the risk of anastomotic failure (Hawley 1973). Several techniques have been discussed to prepare the proximal colon at the time of emergency operation. In the operative theater, antegrade colonic lavage usually meets the problem of solid fecal material. Using this technique in a consecutive series of 93 patients, 71 (47 patients with obstruction and 24 with perforation) underwent resection with primary anastomosis. The following results were reported: operative mortality 8%, clinical anastomotic leak 7%, wound infection 3%, mean duration of hospitalization 13 days (Koruth et al. 1985). To conclude the outlined issues, we would rather recommend a colostomy than establish a primary anastomosis in left-sided ischemic emergencies of the colon.

Small Bowel Emergencies

Ischemia of the small intestine with consecutive morphological changes of the bowel wall always requires the complete resection of the impaired tissue. An end-to-end anastomosis should be established whenever possible. In the case of stoma creation, stoma viability alone may be mis-leading, because more remote areas can be affected by the ischemic process.

Relaparotomy on Demand Versus Planned Relaparotomy

Despite advantages in diagnostic techniques, the decision to reoperate on a critically ill patient ultimately depends on clinical judgement and may be a source of conflict. The clinical scenario of abdominal pain associated with peritoneal signs including tenderness, guarding, and increased abdominal wall tenderness is usually sufficient to diagnose secondary peritonitis. Laboratory data such as C-reactive protein or procalcitonin may support the diagnosis. However, in the clinical setting of an intensive care unit with patients on controlled mechanical ventilation, decreased level of consciousness due to head injury, patients receiving immunosuppressive drugs or generally immunocompromized patients, e. g., in chronic renal dialysis, clinical signs and laboratory data may not be reliable at all in diagnosing secondary peritonitis requiring reoperation. Diagnostic investigations, such as ultrasound or computed tomography, for the detection of residual infection are often not conclusive or are impossible to perform. Principally, two surgical strategies have been advanced to meet the above outlined challenges: (1) relaparotomy on demand and (2) planned relaparotomy (or Etappenlavage). Both procedures were compared just recently in a non-randomized case-control study (Hau et al. 1995). Thirty-eight patients who underwent planned relaparotomy (PR) were matched with 38 patients undergoing relaparotomy on demand (RD). Overall, there was no significant difference in mortality between the groups. Multiple organ failure and septic complications were more frequent in the group of patients undergoing PR than in those undergoing RD. Although not randomized, this study supports the hypothesis that planned relaparotomy should be applied with more caution. It may be restricted to those patients with an Mannheim peritonitis index greater than 29 (Winkeltau et al. 1996). However, prospective randomized studies are not yet available. Clear established guidelines for most RDs are still lacking. Usually, they are performed on the basis of otherwise unexplained, progressive organ dysfunction or bacteremia (van Goor 1997; Nel et al. 1986; Sinanan et al. 1984; Pitcher and Musher 1982; Ferraris 1983; Polk and Shields 1977; Herbrecht et al. 1984). These relaparotomies are technically difficult to perform, have a high morbidity, and often do not reverse organ dysfunction, even when septic foci are encountered and drained (Marshall and Sweeney 1990). To further improve medical decision making when doing a relaparotomy, Pusajo et al. (1993) have developed an abdominal re-operation predictive index, taking into account that the time elapsing from initial surgery to re-operation in the presence of a septic complication is a crucial factor. The authors could demonstrate that the use of this scoring system enabled them to lower mortality among patients undergoing re-operation. The time elapsing between the first operation and relaparotomy could be reduced, and the length of stay in the intensive care unit could be shortened. Moreover, it was concluded that the systematic application of an index, without disregarding clinical judgement, allows the quality of attention to be improved, the cost to be lowered, and the level of conflicts generated by the difficult decision to perform re-operation to be curtailed. The development of neural net-works will probably solve the problem in the near future more clearly on an individual basis – when performing a second look at secondary peritonitis [www.medan.de].

Second Look at Intestinal Ischemia

On the contrary, the indication for second-look laparotomy after surgery for intestinal ischemia is well established. Regardless of the origin – arterial or venous – and unrelated to the procedure – anastomosis or creation of a stoma – second-look laparotomy is mandatory to ensure bowel viability (Kaleya et al. 1992). At the time of initial laparotomy, bowel segments of marginal viability are often preserved in order to avoid a short bowel syndrome. After revascularization by either embolectomy, thrombectomy, or vascular bypass, the questionable ischemic areas may be salvaged, but they need to be reinspected after 24–48 h. In venous mesenteric thrombosis, even after resection of the affected segment and institution of anticoagulation therapy, the process of venous thrombosis may progress. Therefore, additional resection may be required during the second look. It is important to emphasize that the decision to perform a second-look laparotomy is already made during the initial operation and must then be carried out regardless of the patient's post-operative clinical status. In published reports, less than 10% of patients have undergone a second-look procedure, and bowel resections were performed in 25% of these (Schneider et al. 1994). The widespread use of laparoscopic techniques has also been applied for re-exploration in intestinal ischemia. Eypasch (Eypasch et al. 1992) reported six patients with peritonitis or bowel necrosis at the initial operation who underwent laparoscopic reexploration 96 h after primary laparotomy. Open re-exploration was performed in three patients based on the laparoscopic findings; the other three were clarified by means of the second-look laparoscopy with no adverse outcome. Similar results were reported by MacSweeney (MacSweeney and Postelthwaite 1994), Sackier (Sackier 1992) and Slutzki (Slutzki et al. 1996) and support the feasibility of second-look laparoscopy in patients with mesenteric ischemia (Zamir and Reissman 1998). It is crucial, however, to be aware of the present limitations of experience using this new technique.

Abdominal Compartment Syndrome

The abdominal compartment syndrome is best characterised by adverse physiological effects (renal, pulmonary, cardiovascular) resulting from increased abdominal pressure. Although different grades of the abdominal compartment syndrome have been suggested, it is up to now not clear, which abdominal pressure is required for various adverse events. Thus, it is reported that up to 30% of post-operative general surgery patients have intraabdominal pressures greater than 20 mm Hg, but they do not all have an abdominal compartment syndrome (Sugrue 2000). Obviously, the volume status of the patients plays a pivotal role in this context. Measuring intraabdominal pressure by the intravesical technique may be the best technique to circumvent this problem, but in our experience, the clinical investigation of the patients abdomen is still of utmost importance. Although not supported by randomised controlled trials we believe that in generalised peritonitis a primary closure of the fascia during the first operation is harmful for the patient. We advocate the closure of only the skin, since it is our impression that generalised peritonitis leads via the way of excessive gut swelling to an abdominal compartment syndrome. The latter condition even is accentuated by the high volume therapy when septic shock is present. Alternative surgical techniques for temporary closure of the abdomen are using IV bags, velcro, silicone and zips.

4.3.3.2
Supportive Therapy

A) Hemodynamic Monitoring and Cardiovascular Support

Peripheral arterial vasodilatation and elevation of cardiac output (hyperdynamic phase) are the dominant features of septic shock. These circulatory changes are considered to be the major determinants of tissue oxygen uptake and cellular ischemia, Moreover, disturbances in the microcirculation and peripheral shunting of oxygen have been suggested to be responsible for diminished oxygen extraction and hyperlactataemia in septic shock.

Therefore, it is obvious that hemodynamic monitoring plays a pivotal role in assessing septic shock states.

Methods of hemodynamic monitorings are: arterial blood pressure, central venous pressure, pulmonary artery catheter, fibreoptic pulmonary artery catheter (allowing continous mixed venous oxygen saturation), thermodilution techniques (COLD-monitoring), pulse contour analysis (PICCO-monitoring), trans-oesophageal two-dimensional Doppler ultrasonography (TEE).

Despite the widespread use of the pulmonary artery catheter in critically ill patients there is little evidence that its use is changing the patients` prognosis.

Meanwhile, a consensus conference of the Society of Critical Care Medicine gave the recommendation to organize clinical trials investigating the safety and effectiveness of the pulmonary artery catheter especially in cases of severe sepsis and septic shock (Pulmonary Artery Catheter Consensus Conference 1997).

One of the new technically demanding methods is currently highly disputed: TEE. It can provide valuable informations at the beside about acute cardiac diseases of the critically ill.

Adequate hemodynamic support early in the course of septic shock is of utmost importance.

The following recommendations were given by the Task Force of the American College of Critical Care Medicine, Society of Critical Care Medicine (Task Force of the American College of Critical Care Medicine, Society of Critical Care Medicine 1999):

Basic Principles

1. Patients with septic shock should be treated in an intensive care unit, with continuous electrocardiographic monitoring and monitoring of arterial oxygenation.
2. Arterial cannulation should be performed in patients with shock to provide a more accurate measurement of intra-arterial pressure and to allow beat-to-beat analysis so that decisions regarding therapy can be based on immediate and reproducible blood pressure information.
3. Resuscitation should be titrated to clinical end points of arterial pressure, HR, urine output, skin perfusion, and mental status, and indices of tissue perfusion such as blood lactate concentrations and Svo2.
4. Assessment of cardiac filling pressures may require central venous or pulmonary artery catheterization. Pulmonary artery catheterization also allows

for assessment of pulmonary arterial pressures, cardiac output measurement, and measurement of Svo2.

Fluid Resuscitation

1. Fluid infusion should be the initial step in the hemodynamic support of patients with septic shock. Generation of the hyperdynamic state is dependent on fluid repletion.
2. Initial fluid resuscitation should be titrated to clinical endpoints. Isotonic crystalloids or iso-oncotic colloids may be used for fluid resuscitation. These are equally effective when titrated to the same hemodynamic end points.
3. Invasive hemodynamic monitoring should be considered in those patients not promptly responding to initial resuscitative efforts. Pulmonary edema may occur as a complication of fluid resuscitation and necessitates monitoring of arterial oxygenation. Fluid infusion should be titrated to a level of filling pressure associated with the greatest increase in cardiac output and stroke volume. For most patients, this level will be a pulmonary artery occlusion pressure in the range of 12 to 15 mm Hg.
4. Hemoglobin concentrations should be maintained above 8 to 10 g/dL. In patients with low cardiac output, mixed venous oxygen desaturation, lactic acidosis, widened gastric-arterial PCO_2 gradients, or coronary artery disease, tranfusion to a higher level of hemoglobin may be desired.

Vasopressor Therapy

1. In patients with clinical signs of shock and hypotension not initially responsive to aggressive empiric fluid challenge, dopamine is the first-line agent for increasing blood pressure. Pulmonary artery catheterization is useful to guide therapy.
2. Dopamine and norepinephrine are both effective for increasing arterial blood pressure. It is imperative to ensure that patients are adequately fluid resuscitated. Dopamine raises cardiac output more than norepinephrine, but its use may be limited by tachycardia. Norepinephrine may be a more effective vasopressor in some patients. Phenylephrine is an alternative, especially in the setting of tachyarrhythmias, although experience in patients with septic shock is limited.
3. Epinephrine should be considered for refractory hypotension, although adverse effects are common.
4. Routine administration of low doses of dopamine to maintain renal function is not recommended but low-dose dopamine may increase renal blood flow in some patients when added to norepinephrine.

Inotropic Therapy

1. Dobutamine is the first choice for patients with low cardiac index (<2.5 L/min/m^2) after fluid resuscitation and inadequate MAP. Dobutamine may cause hypotension and/or tachycardia in some patients, especially those with decreased filling pressures.

2. In patients with evidence of tissue hyperperfusion, the addition of dobut-amine may be helpful to increase cardiac output and improve organ perfu-sion. A strategy of routinely increasing cardiac index to predefined "supra-normal" levels (>4.5 L/min/m^2) has not been shown to improve outcome.
3. A vasopressor, such as norepinephrine, and an inotrope, such as dobutamine, can be titrated separately to maintain both MAP and cardiac output.
4. Epinephrine and dopamine can be used to increase cardiac output, but mesenteric perfusion may be decreased with epinephrine, and gastric muco-sal perfusion may be decreased with dopamine.

A practical approach for the treatment of septic shock has been suggested by Martin et al. (2000):

Clinical Parameters

Central Venous Pressure — Fluid Challenge: 5–7 ml/kg of colloid or Crystalloid in 15–20 min

Fluid Challenge Ineffective — 2nd, 3rd Fluid Challenge

Fluid Challenge Failure or Deleterious — Dopamine 7–15 µg/kg/min Echocardiography, P. A. Catheter

Optimal PCWP? (12–15 mm Hg)

Fluid Challenge

Vascular Failure suspected — Myocardial Dysfunction Suspected

CI >3–4 l/min/m^2 — CI <3 l/min/m^2
Svo2 >65–70% — Svo2 <65%
PCWP 12– — PCWP >15 mm Hg

Dopamine
+Norepinephrine 0.5–5 µg/kg/min
(+)Dobutamine 5–20 µg/kg/min
when CI and/or Svo2 decrease
by 15% or more

Dopamine
+Dobutamine 5–20 µg/kg/min
(+)Norepinephrine
0.5–5 µg/kg/min to maintain
meanblood pressure >70 mm Hg

Failure

+ epinephrine 0.5–5 µg/kg/min or
phenylephrine 0.5–5 µg/kg/min

B) Acute Respiratory Distress Syndrome

ARDS (acute respiratory distress syndrome) is characterised by limited pul-monary gas exchange, radiologically visible pulmonary infiltrates, changes in the lung-mechanics and pulmonary hypertension. A non-cardiogenic lung edema is the consequence of the increased permeability of the alveolar capillary mem-branes and the increased pulmonary arterial tension.

A further characteristic symptom is severe hypoxemia which cannot be significantly improved by the raising of FiO_2. The reason for the hypoxemia is the high intrapulmonary right-left shunt showing the perfusion of non-ventilated lung areas.

Any serious illness can principally lead to an acute lung deficiency. But in most cases it is the consequence of direct lung damage such as lung contusion, aspiration of the acidic stomach content, pneumonia, inhalation trauma or indirect lung damage through sepsis, polytrauma, or hypertransfusion. All studies conclude that sepsis is the primary risk factor: 47–63% of all ARDS cases are associated with a sepsis syndrome.

Knowledge of the risk factors and their general importance with respect to ARDS progression led the Consensus Conference (Bernard et al. 1994) to assign direct and indirect risk factors:

Direct risk factors
Aspiration
Diffuse Pneumonia (bacterial, viral etc.)
Irritant gas inhalation
Lung contusion

Indirect risk factors
Sepsis syndrome
Severe extra-thoracic trauma
Hypertransfusion during attempts of resuscitation
Cardiopulmonary Bypass

In addition, this Consensus Conference defined the terms of ARDS and ALI:

ARDS

I.   Acute appearance of pathology
II. Ratio of partial arterial oxygen pressure (PAO_2) to the fraction of inspired oxygen (FiO_2) is less than 200 mm Hg independent of the positive end-expiratory pressure (PEEP) applied.
III. Bilateral infiltrates detected on radiological images of the thorax (ap).
IV. Pulmonary capillary wedge pressure (PCWP) of less than 18 mm Hg or absence of any other signs of left atrial hypertension if the PCWP has not been determined.

ALI

I.   Acute appearance of pathology
II. Ratio of partial arterial oxygen pressure (PAO_2) to the fraction of inspired oxygen (FiO_2) is less than 300 mm Hg independent of the positive end-expiratory pressure (PEEP) applied.
III. Bilateral infiltrates detected on radiological images of the thorax (ap).
IV. Pulmonary capillary wedge pressure (PCWP) of less than 18 mm Hg or absence of any other signs of left atrial hypertension if the PCWP has not been determined.

Dependent on the pathogenesis, mortality is still greater than 50% although higher rates of survival have emerged over the past ten years.

The basis of ARDS therapy is controlled ventilation with PEEP. Even if with controlled ventilation, the gas exchange is deteriorating, associated in general with the appearance of dorsobasal pulmonary infiltrates, the possibility of conventional, assisted ventilation will be limited. Besides the increase of PEEP to allow recruitment of lung areas, it is possible to treat this by permissive hypercapnea, inversed-ratio ventilation, side-separated ventilation with selective PEEP or the application of NO; in clinical trials the partial liquid ventilation method has been used. A further means of treatment is kinetic therapy using special rotation beds and ventilation in the abdominal position. All ventilation treatments so far applied have proven unsuccessful in lowering the lethality of ARDS (Artigas et al. 1998).

Therefore a recently published study of the Acute Respiratory Distress Network has attracted a great deal of attention (Acute Respiratory Distress Network 2000). The study's main findings are that the application of a respiratory volume of 6 ml/kg in contrast to 12 ml/kg for patients with acute lung failure led to a decrease in mortality of 22 %. For this reason, the study was published with the results of only 861 random patients in contrast to the usual 1000. It is worthwhile mentioning that in the group with reduced respiratory volume, a higher PEEP was necessary on the 1st and 3rd day of treatment and that the PaO_2 to FiO_2 ratio still remained poor. Despite these initially poor blood gas values, the final therapeutic outcome of this group was improved. This result underscores the importance of protective lung ventilation.

C) Acute Renal Failure

Acute renal failure is common in critically ill patients. It is frequently seen as part of the multi organ failure syndrome especially when sepsis is the underlying disease. Principally, acute renal failure is not the cause of death in intensive care patients, provided that there is no conscious decision not to treat in the face of another non-recoverable disorder.

Criteria for the diagnosis of acute renal failure are

1. Fall in urine volume to less than 500 ml per day.
2. Rising plasma urea and creatinine concentrations.
3. Rising plasma potassium and phosphate plus falling calcium and venous bicarbonate.

Existing guidelines for the management of patients with oliguria or anuria include (Short and Cumming 1999)

1. Assess and correct any respiratory or circulatory impairment.
2. Manage any life threatening consequences of renal dysfunction (hyperkalaemia, salt and water overload, severe uraemia, extreme acidosis).
3. Exclude obstruction of the urinary tract.
4. Establish underlying causes and institute prompt remedial action.

5. Get a drug history and alter prescription appropriately.
6. Be aware that sepsis is the primary cause in surgical intensive care units.

Continuous renal replacement therapy is increasingly being used to treat acute renal failure in critically ill patients. Thus, just recently it could be demonstrated that ultrafiltration at 35 mL/h/kg and 45 mL/h/kg was associated with a significantly lower mortality of 43% and 42% respectively versus a mortality rate of 59% in the ultrafiltration group at 20 mL/h/kg. It is therefore recommended to start continuous haemofiltration early at 2 L per h or more (Ronco et al. 2000).

D) Stress-ulcer Bleeding

In the last fifteen years a decline in the incidence of stress ulcer bleeding has been observed. One recent study reported even a virtual absence of stress-ulceration related bleeding of patients on ICU receiving prolonged mechanical ventilation without any prophylaxis (Zandstra and Stoutenbeek 1994). It is generally believed that this phenomenon is not exclusively related to the widespread use of H_2 receptor antagonists in intensive care units (ICU), but has to be interpreted in association with multiple improvements in anaesthesiological and surgical techniques. Surprisingly, the diminished rate of stress ulcer bleeding had no influence upon the overall mortality of patients on ICU (Schuster 1993). In this context the argument of an increasing effect of H_2 receptor antagonists on the pneumonia rate, one of the leading causes of death on ICU emerged (Tryba et al 1988; Driks et al. 1987). It was discussed that via the route of an elevated gastric pH, followed by bacterial overgrowth and subsequent tracheal aspiration pneumonia would develop (Cook et al. 1991). This assumption, however, is subject to

Table 8. PLACEBO-controlled studies: effect upon pneumonia rate

	n	Patients	Intervention	Pneumonia rate
Cheadle 1985	200	surgical	cimetidine (CIM) double blind	placebo 1.5% CIM 6.5%
Reusser 1989	40	neurosurgical ventilation > 48 h	ranitidine/antacid (RAN)	placebo 38% RAN 36%
Karlstadt 1990	87	surgical/medical	cimetidine (CIM) double blind	placebo 6% CIM 0%
Apte 1992	34	tetanus, tracheotomized	ranitidine (RAN) and/or antacid	placebo 50% RAN 81%
Metz 1993	167	severe head injury	ranitidine (RAN) double blind	placebo 19% RAN 14%
Martin 1993	131	surgical/medical	cimetidine (CIM) double blind	placebo 9% CIM 0%
Ben-Menachem 1994	300	medical	cimetidine (CIM) sucralfate (SUC) single blind	placebo 6% CIM 13% SUC 12%

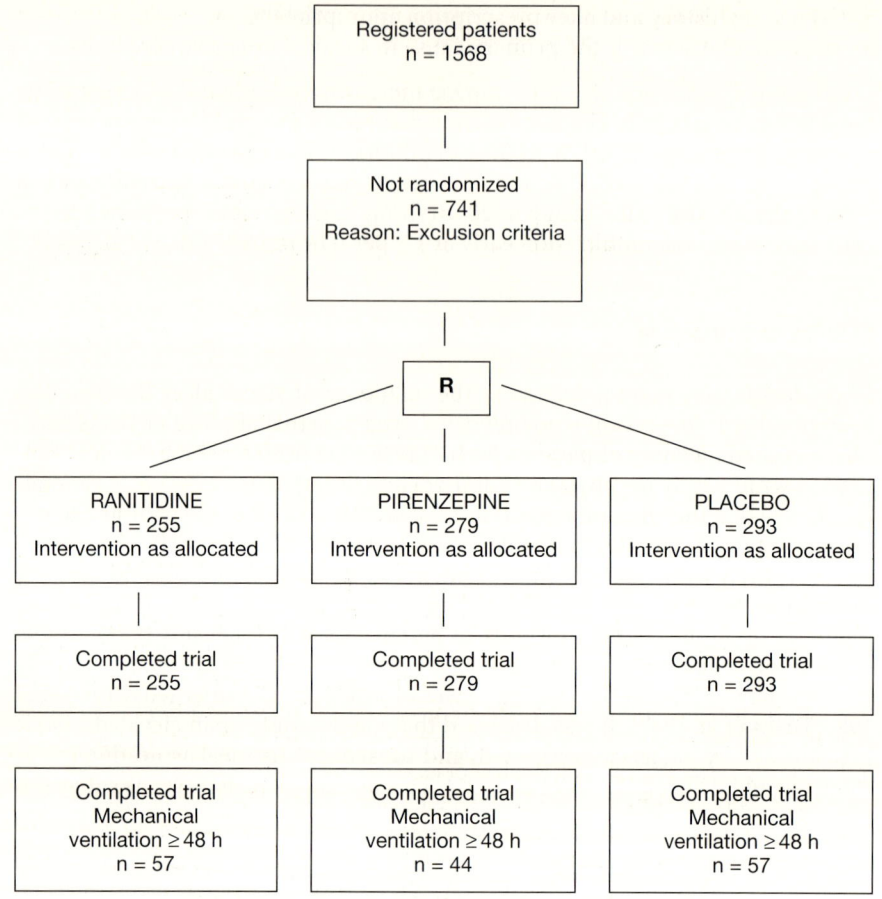

Fig. 8. Trial Profile

controversial discussions. In line with the above outlined hypothesis total gastrectomized patients should develop a very high incidence of pneumonia which is actually not the case. We therefore formulated the hypothesis that stress ulcer prophylaxis with H_2 receptor antagonists does not lead to an increased pneumonia rate. Since only few double blind, placebo controlled trials do exist (for an overview see table 8) with quite differing pneumonia rates and results, patients were randomly assigned to a group with no stress ulcer prophylaxis. The trial considers also pirenzepine which has only minor effects on the gastric pH in comparison with H_2 receptor antagonists (see trial profile fig. 8).

The trial-length was one year. After six months a patient died because of stress ulcer bleeding. At the same time a second patient had stress ulcer bleeding requiring the transfusion of 12 units blood and endoscopic therapy. After breaking the code by the monitor of the study it was evident that the patients belonged to the placebo group (see table 11; patient 7 and 8). Following external

Table 9. General patient characteristics, pneumonia, stress bleeding and mortality (data are means and full range) in patients mechanically ventilated ≥ 48 h

	RANITIDINE	PIRENZEPINE	PLACEBO
PATIENTS (n)	57	44	57
Age (years)	55/22-88	53/18-86	58/22-88
ICU stay (d)	9,7/2-95	9,9/2-39	12,6/2-58[d]
APACHE II	19/2-30	21/12-34	18/1-28
Mechanical ventilation (d)	8,2/2-93	8/2-32	10,2/2-55[c]
Pneumonia (n)[a]	10	10	12
Stress bleeding (n)[b]	3	3	1
Mortality (n)	7	12	12

[a] $\chi^2 = 3{,}55$; DF = 2; p = 0,17;   [b] $\chi^2 = 1{,}79$; DF = 2; p = 0,41;   [c] $\chi^2 = 8{,}54$; DF = 2; p = 0,01; [d] $\chi^2 = 7{,}54$; DF = 2; p = 0,02.

and internal discussions exclusion criteria were extented by postoperative drugs like aspirine, cortisone and coumarine.

Of 827 randomized patients a total of 158 fulfilled the primary study end point mechanical ventilation ≥ 48 h. General patient characteristics, pneumonia, stress bleeding and mortality of these patients are summarized in table 9. There is no statistical difference between the groups with respect to the pneumonia rate. Placebo treated patients had a significantly longer ICU-stay with a concomitant longer mechanical ventilation period.

Stress ulcer bleeding had no serious clinical sequelae in patients with ranitidine (blood transfusions, 2 units each) and pirenzepine (blood transfusion, 4 units each) except in two placebo patients. Both underwent cardiac surgery (aortic valve replacement; bypass-surgery) with postoperative medication of coumarine, aspirine and cortisone, respectively. The first patient died due to his ulcer bleeding, the second one received 12 units of blood. Bleeding had been controlled by endoscopic intervention. After the extension of exclusion criteria no further bleeding was observed in placebo treated patients.

Table 11 summarizes the data of clinical relevant stress ulcer bleeding during the complete trial.

Prophylaxis has unequivocally decreased the formerly frightening stress ulcer bleeding of patients on ICU, although the general mortality of this population could not be reduced. This obvious discrepancy stimulated numerous investigations, and the knowledge of nosocomial infection as critical determinant in this context was established (Tryba 1989). According to this hypothesis the pH-elevating effect of H_2-receptor antagonists is prompting gastric bacterial growth which in turn causes via an oesophageal ascension and subsequent tracheal aspiration more pneumonias. Thus, giving sucralfate, which does not alter gastric pH, yields significantly less pneumonias (Prod'hom et al. 1994). In this prospective randomized study, late pneumonias occurred in a significantly smaller extent in the sucralfate group than in the ranitidine group (5% vs 21%). In a recent study that compared the results of sucralfate versus maximal H_2 blocker infusion therapy plus antacids, the overall pneumonia rate was 27,5% in the H_2 blocker antacid group and 29,8% in the sucralfate group with a significant level of p = 0,48 (Maier et al. 1994.). This study implies a considerable reduction of charges/cost for the sucralfate approach. Contrary to the above mentioned studies, in another randomized trial with trauma patients, no difference could be found (Pickworth et al 1993). Our data, *placebo controlled*, are corroborating these results (Table 9). Furthermore, there are also *placebo controlled* studies in long-term ventilated patients supporting the results of our study. Thus, Reusser et al. randomized 40 neurosurgical patients requiring mechanical ventilation for > 48 h to either a control group receiving no stress-ulcer prophylaxis or to a ranitidine/antacid group. There was no significant difference in the pneumonia rate of patients with and without stress ulcer prophylaxis. In line with these findings Metz et al. (1993) also could not find any difference in 167 placebo controlled randomized patients with severe head injury.

On the contrary, Apte et al. (1992) demonstrated on 34 randomized tracheo-tomized patients with tetanus receiving i. v. ranitidine (50 mg, 6 hourly and/or antacids) or neither ranitidine nor antacids, significant more pneumonias in the ranitidine group (81%) than in the control group (50%) were found. Moreover, patients treated with ranitidine developed pneumonia significantly earlier than patients in control-groups.

With respect to pirenzepine only few trials are available, the largest one having been conducted by Tryba et al. (1988). 400 patients were randomized to a ranitidine (200 mg) or to a pirenzepine (50 mg) group. 8 out of 28 patients on mechanical ventilation receiving ranitidine developed pneumonias (28.6%) versus 3 out of 33 patients on mechanical ventilation under pirenzepine (9.1%) which is statistically significant at a level of p < 0.05. One reason for the striking difference to our results might be the different ranitidine and pirenzepine dosages used.

Finally, the comparable pneumonia rates in our pirenzepine and control-group patients are underlining the knowledge that H_2-receptor antagonists with the dosage used do not increase the pneumonia risk of long-term ventilated patients in critical condition. In agreement with the clinical experience, all patients with pneumonia were associated with a prolonged ventilation. In addition, confounding parameters like nasogastric tubes and tracheostomas are obviously of no statistical relevance in this context (Table 10).

Table 10. Nasogastric tube (NGT duration > 48 h, duration > 4 days; n = number of patients) and tracheostoma (n) in patients mechanically ventilated ≥ 48 h

	RANITIDINE	PIRENZEPINE	PLACEBO
NGT > 48 h; n	53	42	55
NGT > 4 d; n	20	26	35
Tracheostoma; n	8	7	13

Table 11. Synopsis of clinical relevant bleeding

	RANITIDINE	RANITIDINE	RANITIDINE	PIRENZEPINE	PIRENZEPINE	PIRENZEPINE	PLACEBO	PLACEBO
Diagnosis	Ileus	Polytrauma	Carcinoma of the floor of the mouth, liver cirrhosis	Coronary heart disease	Head trauma	Polytrauma	Aortic valve disease	Coronary heart disease
Mechanical Ventilation (d)	12	12	2	13	29	18	1	4
Day of bleeding postop	21	10	9	24	21	10	12	13
Mortality	Death at 43th day postop	Survivor	Survivor	Survivor	Survivor	Death at 31th day postop	Death at 12th day postop	Survivor

Especially in view of the pneumonia problem and the costs the question for or against a general stress ulcer prophylaxis dominates the discussion. Accordingly, high risk groups should be defined whether receiving prophylaxis or not. Thus, Cook et al. (1994) could demonstrate in a large prospective multicenter trial that the independent risk factors, controlled ventilation for more than 48 h and coagulopathy (platelets < 50000, prothrombin time $> 1^1/_2$ of normal value or partial thromboplastin time > 2 times of normal value), predetermine for stress ulcer bleeding. In this non-randomized study, collegues were encouraged to withhold prophylaxis. Patients with CNS trauma, burns more than 30 % of the body surface and organ transplantations were given prophylaxis a priori. Comparing the results of Cook (Cook et al. 1994) with our data, some coincidence is apparent. In general, only patients mechanically ventilated for more than 48 h were bleeding. However, two patients were ventilated only 1 and 2 days, respectively, only two patients experienced a coagulopathy. Moreover, a crucial point remains unsettled: the above mentioned risk factors may evolve only during the course of an ICU-stay – is it then too late to start with stress ulcer prophylaxis?

A main finding marking the course of our study was the death of a patient directly related to bleeding. Unrevealing the code showed that the patient belonged to the placebo group. At the same time, a second patient had to be transfused with 12 units blood due to stress bleeding. Fortunately, endoscopic intervention was successful. Since both patients had coumarine and aspirine as well as cortisone postoperatively, the consensus after controversial discussions was to extend exclusion criteria; i.e. patients after cardiac and vascular surgery were no longer considered for randomization. These patients (n = 510) were prophylactically treated with H_2 receptor antagonists and demonstrated no evidence for clinical relevant stress bleeding. From that time on no further bleeding could be observed in patients treated with placebo.

Although it is intriguing to speculate that in the defined randomized population there are apparently no differences between the groups with respect to clinical relevant stress bleeding, it is evident from the bleeding rates in patients on prolonged mechanical ventilation, that about 3000 patients would be needed to detect a 30–40 % decrease in bleeding. Thus, only a multicenter trial can solve this issue whether stress ulcer prophylaxis is necessary or not. Our sample size is too small to allow any definite conclusion about this question.

Accordingly, the results of this study are to same extent contrary to the findings of a recent meta-analysis (Cook et al 1996) indicating that histamine-2-receptor antagonists may be associated with an increased incidence of pneumonia. Most important, the authors found that sucralfate was associated with a trend towards a lower rate of pneumonia when compared with other antacids or histamine-2-receptor antagonists. They also found a trend towards reduced mortality when sucralfate was compared with histamine-2-receptor antagonists and a significant reduction when it was compared with antacids. But, as was pointed out by the authors, further studies (i.e. multicenter studies with recruitment of thousands of patients) are needed whether these figures are real.

In conclusion, we can demonstrate that in surgical critical ill patients on mechanically ventilation for ≥ 48 h stress ulcer prophylaxis with H_2-receptor antagonists pneumonia rate is not adversely affected.

E) The Icteric Critically Ill Patient

The icterus of the intensive care patient can pose problems in differential diagnosis. A clear analysis of the pathogenesis is in most cases impossible due to multiple concomitant and overlapping mechanisms. The primary causes are an increased bilirubin level and a simultaneously decreased hepatic excretion capacity caused by blood transfusion, hematoma resorption, shock or sepsis. Very differing prognoses have been reported for post-surgical icteric patients. It is, however, commonly agreed that a progressive icterus can forewarn a lethal progression.

The occurrence of icterus after large-scale surgery was observed as early as at the beginning of this century (Guthrie 1903). After the introduction of halothane narcosis in the fifties, the interest in understanding the correlation increased. Very different frequencies of post-surgical icterus are reported, thus an increase in bilirubin levels was found in 44 of 143 patients undergoing abdominal or thoracic surgery or that of the extremities within the first week after intervention (Herfarth and Körner 1965). The difficulty in analysing these cases by differential diagnosis is seen in 29 of the cases in which the etiologically remained unclear. Other authors report frequencies of post-surgical icterus after elective, abdominal surgery of less than 1% (Clarke et al 1976) and of 2.4% (Schriefers and Wenn 1967). From this last report, it can be unambiguously concluded that the severity of the surgical intervention and the post-surgical complications profoundly influence the bilirubin values: icterus was observed with a frequency of 23.5% after bi-cavity intervention, 11% after stomach surgery and 23% after relaparotomy due to post-surgical complication. The frequency of relaparotomy is also associated with a high incidence of icterus in our patients (Table 12). The frequency of icterus also corresponds to the mode of admission of the patients, this being 24% for emergency versus 4.9% for elective admissions (Table 13).

Table 12. Frequency of re-interventions and hyperbilirubinemia (Lit)

Number of re-operations	Patients n (%)	Death n (%)	Icterus n (%)	Icterus + Death n
1	86 (70.5)	13 (15.1)	27 (31.4)	11
2	23 (18.9)	8 (34.8)	11 (47.8)	4
3	6 (5)	2 (33.3)	5 (83.3)	1
4	2 (1.6)	2 (100)	2 (100)	2
5	2 (1.6)	1 (50)	1 (50)	1
6	2 (1.6)	1 (50)	2 (100)	1
7	1 (0.8)			
Total	122	25 (20.5)	48 (39.3)	20

Table 13. Mode of admission and hyperbilirubinemia (Lit)

	Total n (%)	Death n (%)	Icterus n (%)	Icteris + Death n
Elective Admissions	1096 (86.0)	33 (3.0)	54 (4.9)	15
Emergency Admissions	179 (14.0)	23 (12.8)	43 (24.0)	13

Table 14. Distribution of the icteric cohort on the surgical services (Lit)

	n	Bilirubin ≥ 2 mg/dl n (%)
Accident Surgery	120	9 (7.5)
Polytrauma	34	14 (41.2)
Vascular Surgery	105	13 (12.4)
Thoracic Surgery	65	2 (3.1)
Cardiac Surgery	617	44 (7.1)
General Surgery	197	12 (6.1)
Urology	94	2 (2.1)
Mandibular Surgery	38	1 (2.6)
Others	5	0

Table 15. Maximal bilirubin values of the icteric patients with respect to the time of hospitalisation and mortality (Lit)

Max. Bilirubin (mg/dl]	n	Day (x/range)	Death (n)
4	64	5.8 (2–19)	13
6	11	11.2 (3–33)	6
8	7	13 (5–26)	3
10	4	11.3 (4–17)	2
15	5	13.2 (5–20)	3
20	4	17.8 (17–209)	3
30	1	25	1
> 30	1	14	1

Increased values of bilirubin are reported following cardiological surgery in 23% of all cases (Chu et al. 1987). This is not entirely in accordance with our experience. Following cardiological operations we observe an increase in bilirubin in only 7.1% of all cases; this constitutes a frequency similar to that seen for patients in general surgery (Table 14). In a general way, three forms of post-surgical icterus are known (Banks et al. 1982; Hawker 1991): 1. Hyper-production of bilirubin, 2. Hepato-cellular damage, 3. Extra-hepatic biliary obstruction (this last form is not being dealt with in this study). A hyper-production of bilirubin is classically caused by the hemolysis of transfused blood and by the resorption of blood (hematoma, free intra-luminal blood). Hepato-cellular dysfunction is caused by hypotension, hypoxemia, medication and sepsis. It should be pointed out that two pathological processes occur in the case of hepato-cellular damage:

symptoms resembling hepatitis and intra-hepatic cholestase (Becker and Lamont 1988; Hawker 1991). The hepatitis-like process is characterised by an increase in transaminase whereas the levels of alkaline phosphatase increase only slightly. This combination was not found within our cohort. The intra-hepatic cholestase level, which exhibits a similar enzyme pattern to extra-hepatic obstruction, can be associated with significant increases in alkaline phosphatase whereas transaminase values are generally only slightly raised. These requirements tend to correspond better to our results although the incidence of increased alkaline phosphatase levels did not reach significant values in our group of icteric patients. The symptoms of post-surgical, intra-hepatic cholestase, first described by Caroli et al. (1950) and further characterised by Schmidt et al. (1965) through the term "benign post-surgical intra-hepatic cholestase", usually start within a few days of surgical intervention reaching a peak at the end of the second week (see also Table 15).

Pathologically relevant factors (Table 16) are the increased administration of blood, the incidence of shock as well as septic phenomena (MOF, SOF). Since a normal liver is capable of metabolising ca. 250 ± 350 mg bilirubin per day, the rapid transfusion of several units of blood can rapidly exceed the liver's capacity to metabolise bilirubin, especially in cases of shock. Besides this, the resorption of a hematoma (500 ml of blood results in ca. 2500 mg bilirubin) constitutes an additional burden. The latter observation possibly explains the frequency of hyper-bilirubinemia in cases of polytrauma (Table 14) and is in agreement with observations made by others (Maier et al. 1994).

Furthermore, the icterus can be the only sign of an extra-hepatic infection (i.e. sepsis) in critically ill patients (Brooks et al. 1991). Accordingly, Banks et al. found an icterus in 63% of patients with septic shock and Miller et al. reported that severe bacterial infections associated with an icterus result in a mortality of 43%. If serum bilirubin does not decrease upon adequate antibiotic treatment, the prognosis is considered to be very poor. In the study of Franson (Franson et al. 1989), all of the patients died under circumstances similar to the above.

Table 16. Non-icteric and icteric patients – Pathophysiologically relevant data (mean values/ range) (Lit)

	Total group	non-icteric patients	Bilirubin (2mg/dl)
Ventilation [days]	2 (0–58)	1.3 (0–32)	12.5 (1–58)*
APACHE-Score	17.6 (0–37)	17.5 (0–37)	18.7 (0–34)*
MOF-Score [9]	2.8 (0–12)	2.5 (0–12)	6.6 (1–12)*
SOF-Score [7,13]	6.3 (0–28)	5.8 (0–20)	12.6 (3–28)*
EC (n)	3.3 (0–85)	2.4 (0–47)	13.5 (0–85)*
Shock period (n)	0.1 (0–10)	0.1 (0–8)	0.9 (0–10)*
CVT [cm H_2O]	9.8 (0–30)	9.1 (0–30)	17.6 (8–30)*
PEEP [mm Hg]	1.7 (0–25)	1.3 (0–25)	7.2 (0–20)*

* $p < 0,05$.
MOF = "multi organ failure"; SOF = "sepsis organ failure"; EC = Erythrocyte concentration; CVT = central venous tension; PEEP = positive end expiratory pressure; Shock period = systolic blood tension; < 90 mm Hg for at least 2 h with historically documented hypotension being excluded.

Table 17. Frequency and date of deaths among the icteric and non-icteric cohort

Date of death	Total group n (%)	icteric cohort n (%)	non-icteric cohort n (%)
1 – 4	24 (42.9)	18 (64.3)	6 (21.4)
5 – 8	9 (16.1)	5 (17.9)	4 (14.3)
9 – 12	4 (7.1)	1 (3.6)	3 (10.7)
13 – 16	8 (14.3)	3 (10.7)	5 (17.9)
> 16	11 (19.6)	1 (3.6)	10 (35.7)

Although mortality was significantly higher in our group of icteric patients in comparison to the non-icteric cohort, we note that a post-surgical intra-hepatic cholestase is not of importance in itself. Calculations of the indices for sensitivity, specificity, positive and negative predictive values with respect to the criteria for survival or non-survival in the case of a bilirubin cut-off value of > 6 mg %, support this opinion and correspond to that of other authors (te Brekhorst et al 1988). The decisive factor for mortality is the underlying pathogenesis, which for the critically ill patient is almost exclusively found to be sepsis and multi-organ dysfunction. This becomes clearer with the very high SOF- and MOF-score values of icteric patients (Table 16). This is also reflected by when death occurs: 64.3 % of the deaths within the icteric group occurred on the 1st – 4th day, versus day 17.9 among the non-icteric patients (Table 17). Significantly, although mortality was 29 %, the APACHE II score of this cohort was not increased.

4.4
Case Discussion (Two Patients with Septic Shock from the MEDAN Project www.medan.de)

A)

A 64-year old man underwent a residual gastrectomy because of a signet-ring cell carcinoma.

Physical examination (first day in the intensiv care unit):
Temperature: 36,4 °C
Pulse: 110
Blood Pressure: 160/90
General: Height 169 cm, Weight 69 kg
Chest: pleural effusion left > right (not necessary to puncture)
Abdomen: smooth, florid meteorism

Laboratory findings:

	Leukocyte ×1000/µl	CRP mg/l	Erythrocyte ×1000000/µl	Hb mg/dl	Hkt %	Thrombocyte ×1000/µl	Fibrinogen mg/dl	TPZ %
Normal	4.3–10 ×1000/µl	<0.8 mg/dl	4.4–5.9 ×1000000/µl	14–18 mg/dl	42–52%	140–440/µl	150–450 mg/dl	70–120
Day in ICU								
1	23.1		3.45	10.3	31	215	424	64
10	13	20.2	3.87	11.2	34.4	357	746	71
12	20.4	16.8	3.68	7.5	35	127	231	52
13	16.7	22.6	3.58	8.8	28.6	58	304	58
15	19.1	20.5	3.66	10.5	32	100	446	65
20	32.29	3.1	3.94	11.1	34.4	512	379	74

	PTT sec	TZ sec	AT III %	GOT U/l	GPT U/l	GGT U/l	CHE kU/l	Lactate mg/dl
Normal	35–55 sec	14–21 sec	80–120 %	<18 U/l	<22 U/l	<28 U/l	3–8 kU/l	0.63–2.44 mmol/l
Day								
1	42.3		47	10				17
10	41	11	82	39	31	92	1.211	37
12	38.5	13	69	25	16	52	0.907	60
13	40.6	11	71	13	11	33	1.318	36
15	38.8		61	10				20
20	50.1	19	70	10	8	48	1.892	13

	Amylase U/l	Lipase U/l	Krea mg/dl	Kalium mmol/l	Natrium mmol/l	BZ mg/dl
Normal	<120 U/l	<190 U/l	0.84–1.36 mg/dl	3.6–5.4 mmol/l	134–150 mmol/l	70–100 mg/dl
Day						
1	17		0.8	3.8	146	165
10	157	203	1.5	3.9	148	184
12	81	81	1	3.8	152	333
13	54		0.8	4.2	150	211
15	17		0.6	3.8	148	209
20	202	138	0.6	4.4	137	132

Medical history:
The patient is in state after a Billroth's operation II because of an ulcer 43 years ago. He had a cholecystectomy nine years ago.

Hospital course:
He underwent a residual gastrectomy because of a signet-ring cell carcinoma of the stomach, a splenectomy and a lymphadenectomy. He was brought to the intensive care unit (ICU) with a partial respiratory failure. The patient was extubated and then breathing spontaneously with continuous positive airway pressure (CPAP). He was tachycardiac (100 beats/min) and received 12 liters oxygen.

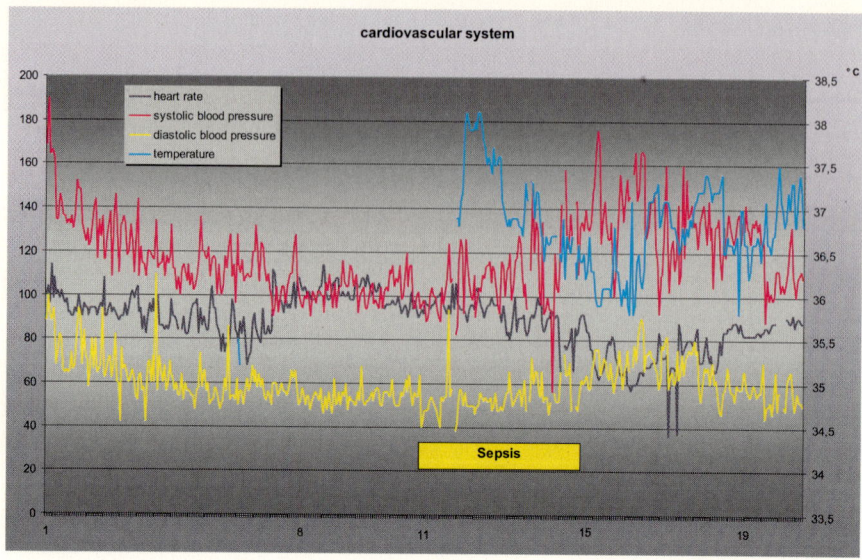

The patient stayed in the ICU for 20 days. Most of the time he was breathing spontanously with an oxygen supply between 4 and 15 liters. For 6 days he needed to be intubated and received continuous and intermittent positive pressure ventilation (CPPV respectively IPPV) on the 12th day of his stay in the ICU. From the 13th to the 16th day he was breathing with biphasic positive airway pressure (BIPAP) and on the 17th day he was ventilated with synchronized intermittent mandatory ventilation (SIMV) before he got extubated. He was ventilated with a positive endexspiratory pressure (PEEP) between 5 and 7 cm H_2O.

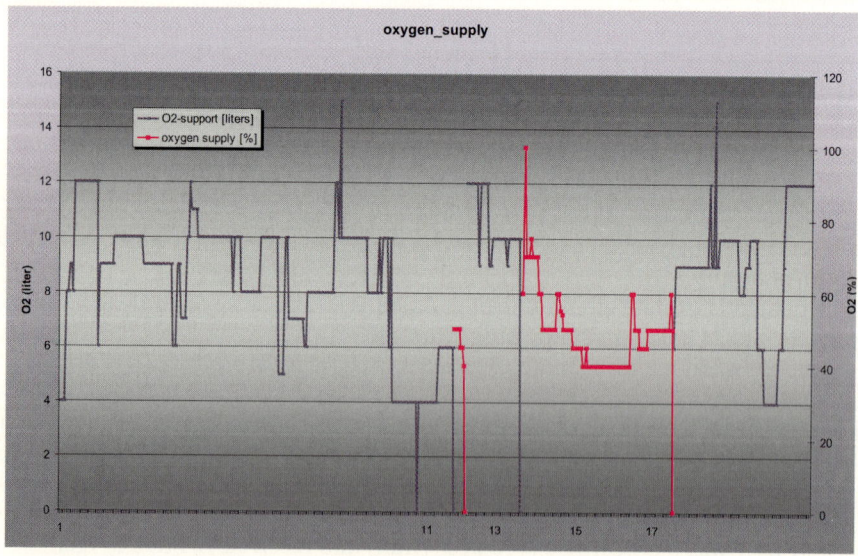

The next graphic shows the fluid balance. The patient received Pentaglobin® for three days. He got a perfusor with 33,3 ml/h for 3 hours and for the rest of the three days it ran with 14 ml/h. In the graphic below Pentaglobin-Volume is included in the fluid supply.

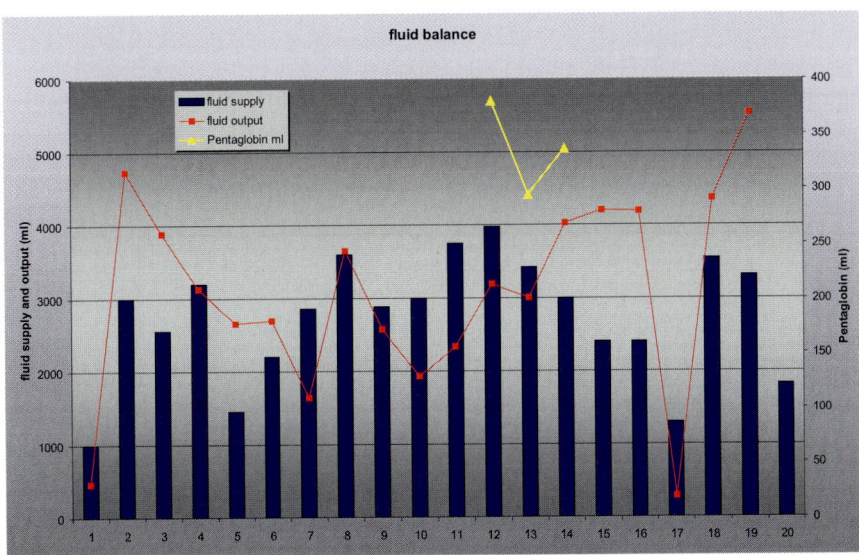

He showed the criterions of systemic inflammatory response syndrome (SIRS) from the 1st until the 15th day. He was tachycardic from the 1st to the 14th day and had a leukocytosis at all of the 20 days except from the 3rd until the 5th day. During the first ten days the results of the microbiologic swab of his nose, the central venous catheter tip and the culture of catheterurine was negative. At the 11th day there was found plenty of methicillin resistent Staphylococcus aureus (MRSA), moderate Stenotrophomonas maltophilia and little Candida species in the abdominal swab. The swab of the nose was still negative. Two days later plenty of MRSA was found in the patients nose and moderate Candida species. Abdominally there was now moderate MRSA and plenty of Stenotrophomonas maltophilia. At the 16th day his catheterurine and the central venous catheter tip was negative, in his nose was only a little Candida and no MRSA, but in the tracheal secretion was a little MRSA. So he fulfilled the criterions of sepsis from the 11th until the 15th day.

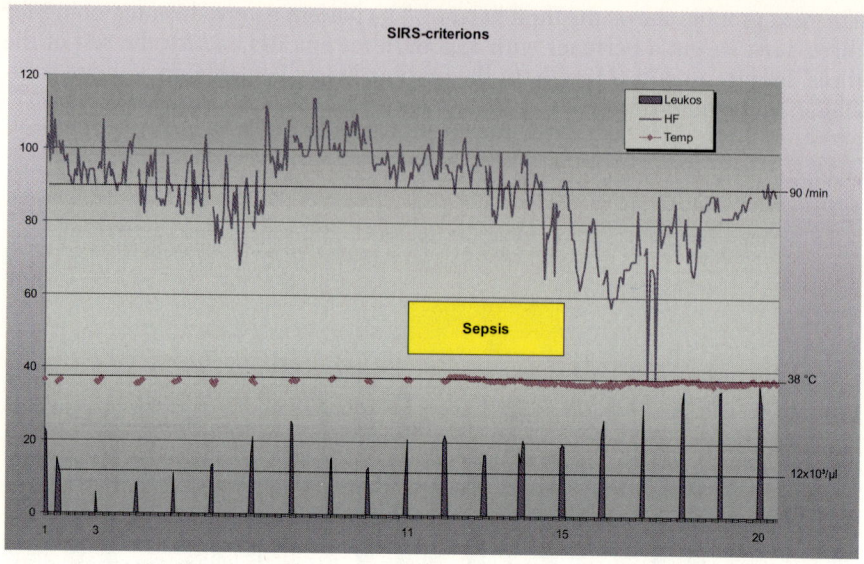

He received low dose dopamine during his stay in the ICU. At the 12th and 14th day he needed higher dose of dopamine, because he was in septic shock. A single dose of epinephrine about 10 µg was given at the 14th day.

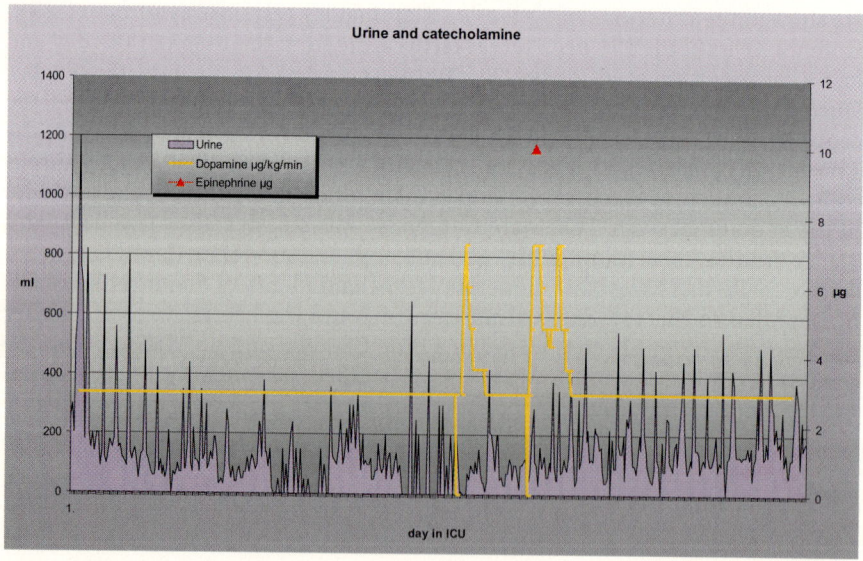

He got a daily dose furosemide between 30 and 120 mg.

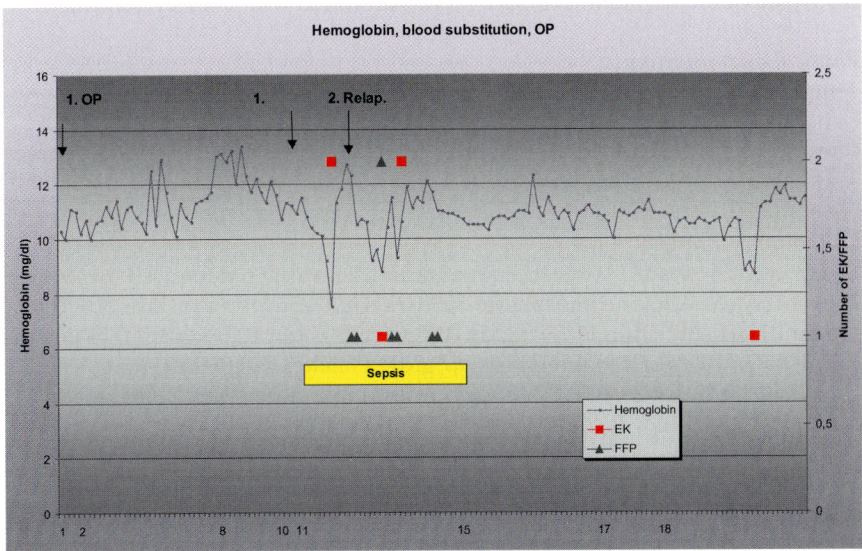

The patient underwent an operation which was a residual gastrectomy combined with splenectomy and lymphadenectomy. On the 11th ICU day it was necessary to operate him again, because of an anastomotic leak of the esophagojejunostomy and an intraabdominal abscess. His preoperatively lactat rose up to 60mmol/l. He received a lavage and a drainage. Intraoperative he was stable and he needed no foreign blood. Two days later another relaparotomy was performed oversuturing the anastomotic leak of the esophagojejunostomy. Intraoperatively a serious purulent peritonitis was found and a swab was taken. On the next day the patient was separated because of MRSA. After 20 days in the ICU he was transferred to a surgical ward.

Critical Comment

Breakdown of the esophagojejunal anastomosis is a serious complication following total gastrectomy. Depending upon the extent of the leak it is usually necessary to perform a relaparotomy establishing a complete new anastomosis. Smaller leaks may be managed conservatively using interventional techniques. In the present case during the first relaparotomy only the abscess was drained without clearing the sepsis source: the anastomotic leakage; thus, in a second relaparotomy this was done by an oversuture. At the same time, a serious purulent peritonitis was present, indicating a lethal challenge for the patient. He finally survived with no further surgical intervention (Etappenlavage, relaparotomy on demand), intriguing to speculate that the patient had profited by the Pentaglobin therapy.

B)

A 73-year-old male, jaundiced patient, was admitted with cholecystolithiasis.

Physical examination:
Temperature: 36,5°C; Pulse 88/min; Blood pressure 210/90 mm Hg
General: Height 176 cm; Weight 94 kg
Chest: breath sounds normal
Abdomen: painless, tender

Laboratory findings:
Electrolytes: Sodium 141 mval/L; Potassium 4,0 mval/L; Calcium 4,3 mval/L;
Liver enzymes: Alkaline phosphates 805 U/L; GGT 255 U/L; Amylase 21 U/L;
Lipase 10 U/L; Bilirubin 17,59 mg/dL; White cells count 12,6 ×10*6/dL; Red cells
count 3,56 ×105/dL; Haemoglobin 10,7 g/dL; Platelets 174 000/dL;
Coagulation: Quick 59%; PTT 40 sec; Prothrombin time 15 sec.; Fibrinogen 427
mg/dL; AT3 7 U/ml; Glucose 140 mg/dL; Protein 4,4 g/dL.

Medical history:
Allergy, coronary heart disease, left ventricular hypertrophy, hypertension.

Hospital course:
The patient was operated and underwent a cholecystectomy on the 1. day. The
common bile duct was revised and a papillotomy with biopsy was sent for pathology. Postoperatively the patient was brought to the ICU for one night. The
pathological findings confirmed an adeno-carcinoma of the papilla vateri and
the distal common bile duct. On the 2. day the patient underwent a Whipple's
procedure for pancreatic carcinoma. After 7 days recovery in the ICU he was
transferred to a surgical ward for further rehabilitation.

Laboratory

Days in ICU	Platelets 10*6/dL	Prothrombin Time /sec	CRP mg/L	Haemoglobin g/dL	Red cell-concentrate/ml
10.	186000	40	10	14.1	
	132000	33			
11.	91000	32	137	11	
	62000				
	34000				
12.				11.7	
13.				10.6	
14.	25000	30	205	9.1	580
		36			
15.				9.9	280
16.	11000	35		9.9	
17.	19000	33	143	9.3	
18.	16000	22		8.6	280

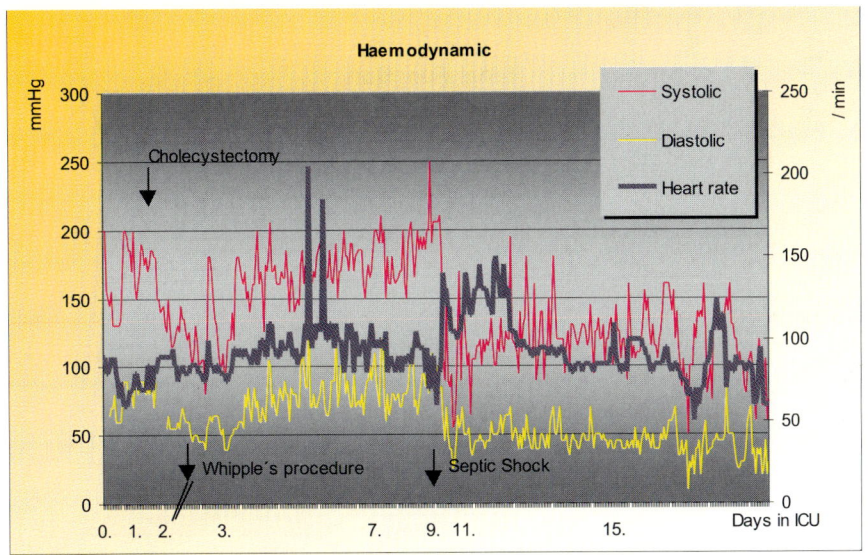

During the first night on the ward on the 10th day, he complained about acute respiratory insufficiency with signs of septic shock. In the ICU he was intubated and ventilated with BIPAP/ASB, sedated (Fentanyl, Brevimytal) and treated with catecholamines (Arterenol, Dobutrex), antibiotics (Clont, Zienam) and catheter in the artery pulmonalis. He developed an anuria, which was treated with diuretics (Lasix), plasmapheresis and later on with haemofiltration (CVVH).

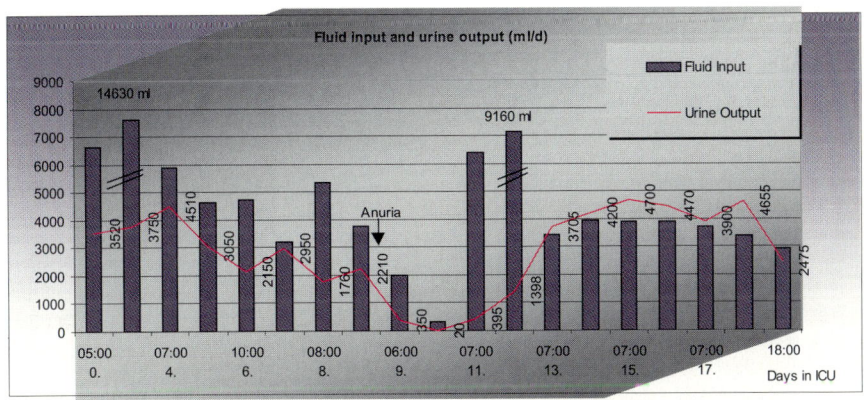

Simultaneously plasma creatinine and urea increased over the normal range-level, as urine secretion decreased on the same day.

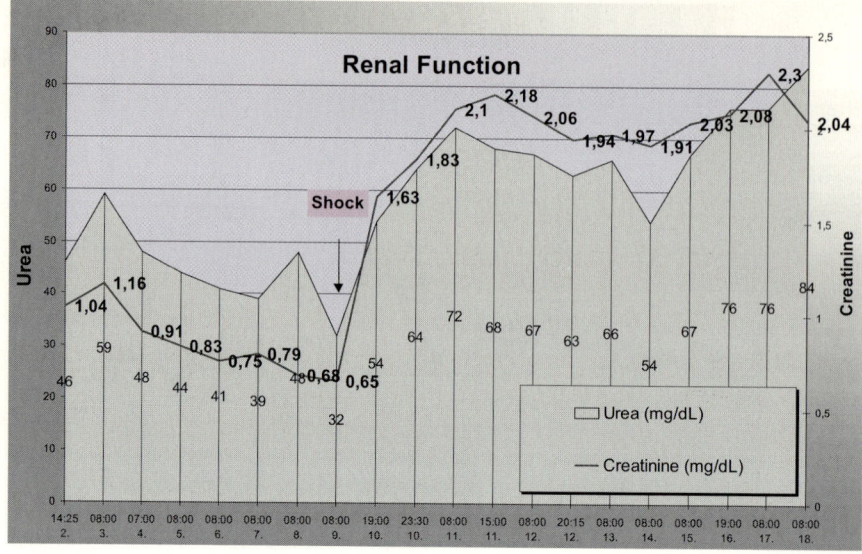

The abdomen CT scan showed paracolon and pararenal exudation and ascites around spleen and liver.

Catecholamines could stabilise perfusion with slight improvement. Therefore catecholamines were reduced on the 14. day and changed with Suprarenin.

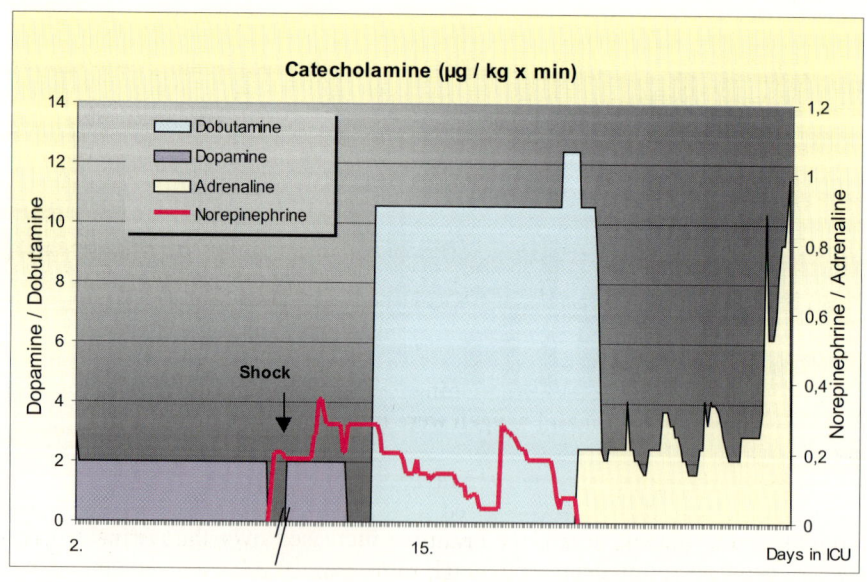

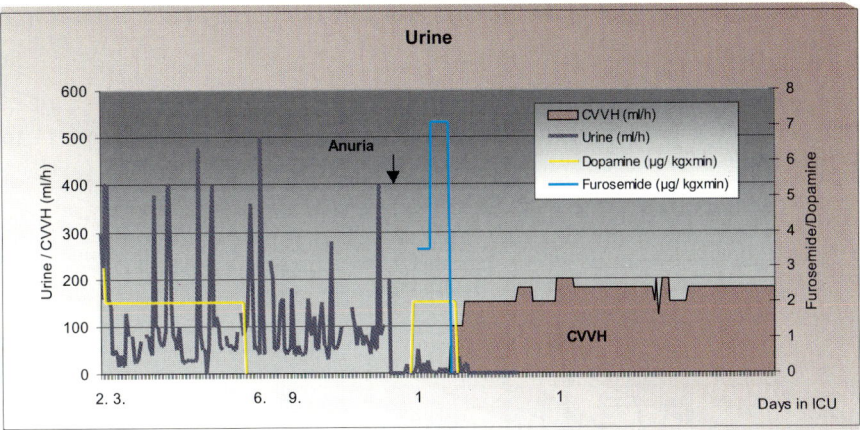

On the 16. day he underwent a tracheotomy for long-term ventilation. He developed thrombopenia, which was successfully substituted with 10,000 ml of eight platelet concentrates.

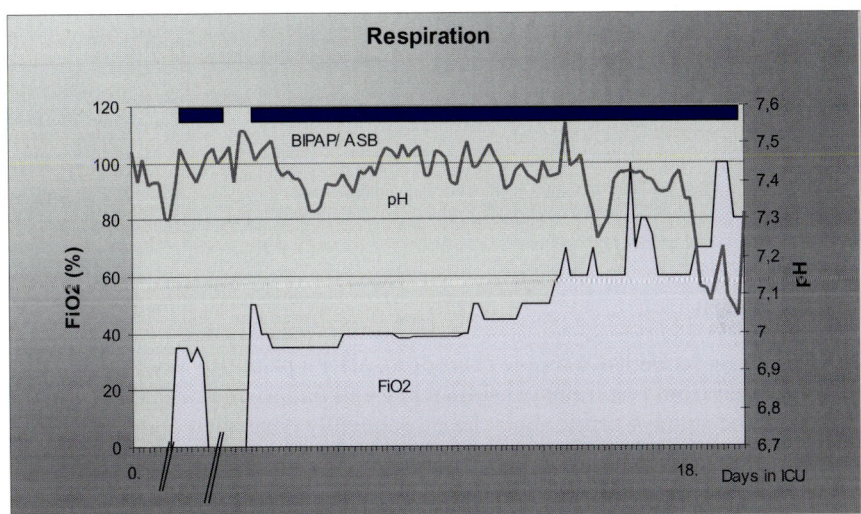

Still the blood gas values were worsening and particularly the haemodynamics kept unstable. Suprarenin and oxygen were increased on high level until the last day (18. day).

On the 16. day ultrasound showed no abdominal abscess.

On the 18. day the patient suffered a severe metabolic acidosis, which was treated with sodium-carbonate and ventilation of 100% oxygen. But still his condition could not be improved although he was given adequate treatment. The

patient died in the night of the 18. day caused by multiorgan-failure and severe
sepsis.

Pentaglobin-Therapy:
Pentaglobin was given in the ICU over 7 days from 10. to 12. day and from 14. to
17. day. Daily dose was between 165 ml to 370 ml.

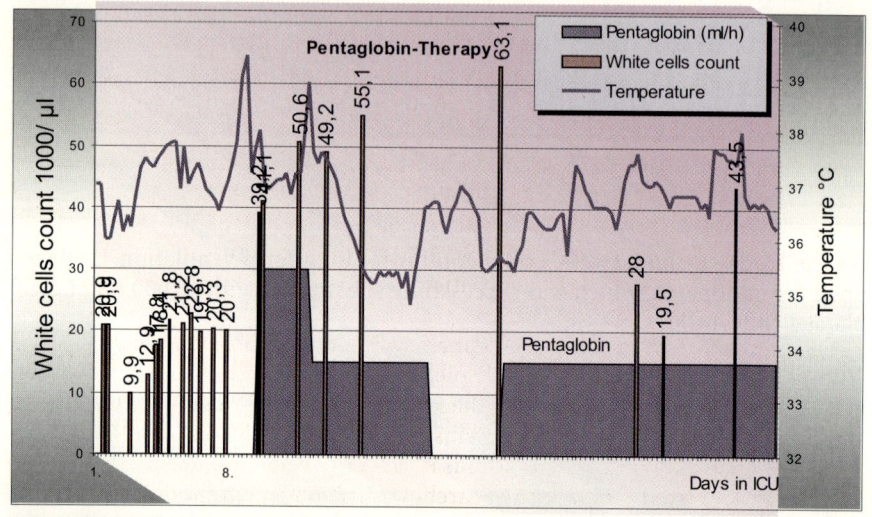

Autopsy:
Necrotising pancreatitis.

Critical Comment

The patient underwent a Whipple procedure. After a primarily uneventful course he suffered from respiratory insufficiency and had to be retransferred to the
ICU. With the signs of septic shock he subsequently developed multi organ failure. Although diagnostic findings (CT, ultrasonography) gave no hints of a sepsis source, following a Whipple procedure one should be highly suspicious of
a breakdown of the pancreatico-jejunostomy. Thus, at least in retrospect and
knowing the autopsy finding, a relaparotomy had been indicated in this case
ruling out this possibility. Without eliminating the sepsis source, even the best
supportive therapy finally fails.

4.5
Cutting Edge Debate

4.5.1
Why Sepsis Trials are Condemned to Fail – Analysing the Heterogeneity of Sepsis Therapy

Since the description of sepsis by Schottmüller (Schottmüller 1914) in 1914, the knowledge regarding the pathophysiology underlying sepsis has substantially increased. Although it has not been possible until now to significantly reduce the mortality of septic shock (Bone 1996; Marshall 2000), which, is as high as 50–60% worldwide.

It is presumed that the number of sepsis cases will further increase. In the USA it is estimated that there will be 400,000 sepsis patients per year (MMWR 1990). Berger (Berger and Beger 1991) calculates that about 20–40% of sepsis patients progress into a septic shock. Assuming a mortality rate of 50%, this means the death of 40,000 to 80,000 patients as a result of septic shock in the USA per year.

There is still no sufficient explanation for the reasons why septic shock occurs, even though more and more pieces of the endogenous mediator system are being identified. This is one of the reasons for the failure of studies dealing with sepsis therapy. The main problems in sepsis therapy are the heterogeneity of the patient groups and the variations in therapy strategies. The meeting of the Lucerne Study Group on Sepsis Research in Marburg in January 1997, featuring experts from 24 centers in Europe, Israel and the USA, demonstrated there is great deal of heterogeneity in patient samples, their diagnosis, and the management of postoperative abdominal sepsis (Encke et al. 1997). In the present study, the therapeutic heterogeneity of septic shock of abdominal origin was analyzed with the aid of algorithms.

An algorithm for 84 selected patients was developed with the help of the computer program ALGO v. 5.1 (Sitter et al. 1999), fulfilling the Consensus-Conference (American College of Chest Physicians/Society of Critical Care Medicine Consensus Conference 1992) criteria for septic shock, this algorithm documents the most important decisions and surgical interventions.

A clinical algorithm is a step-by-step procedure with a defined number of stages in order to find a solution to a clinical problem; this is usually represented in a graphic format. The nomenclature of clinical algorithms used by the computer program ALGO is approved by the Committee on Standardization of Clinical Algorithms of the Society for Medical Decision Making (Society of Medical Decision Making 1992). Three graphically symbolized logical elements were used to describe the algorithms. These are logically connected by if/then commands (fig. 9).

As a first step, three kinds of decisions were made in order to structure the algorithms, these were: 1. Is there a medical indication for a second surgical intervention? 2. Has the condition of the patient changed in such a way that he can be transferred to hospital ward, or does he have to reenter intensive care

| Clinical state box (contains a diagnosis or a defined clinical condition) | Actionbox (contains an activity (eg. operation, transfer to a hospital ward etc.) | 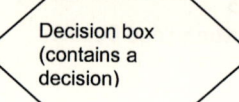 Decision box (contains a decision) |

Fig. 9. Introduction to the symbols used in the algorithms

after having already being dismissed from the intensive care unit and 3. did the patient die?

Taking these criteria into account, the description of the therapy plan in the simplest case can be derived as an algorithm as depicted in figure 10. This example follows a patient with oesophageal carcinoma after resection of the oesophagus, as the patient was stable and no further surgical intervention was required, he was transferred to hospital ward. The fact that complex algorithms can still arise, even with a limitation to basic questions, is demonstrated in figure 11. This case is a description of a patient with a perforating *sigma diverticulitis*, who had undergone a sigma resection; a left hemicolectomy became necessary due to complications. Repeated abdominal lavages were conducted during stationary care, however, the patient eventually died of septic shock.

In the next stage, all patients with an indication for hemofiltration were included in the algorithms. To describe the structural differences in the treatments,

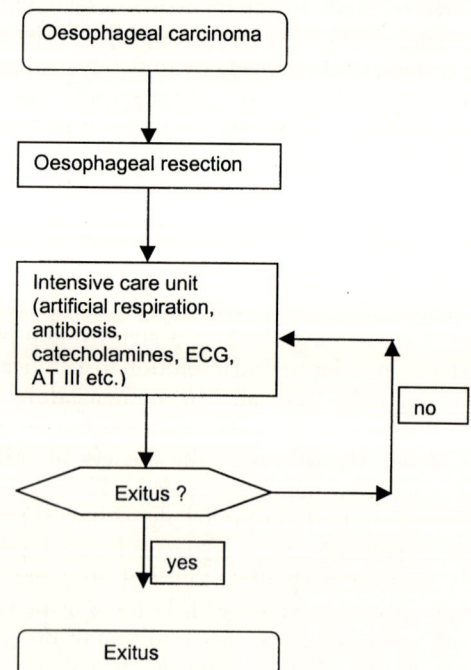

Fig. 10. Algorithm for an oesophageal carcinoma patient with no complications

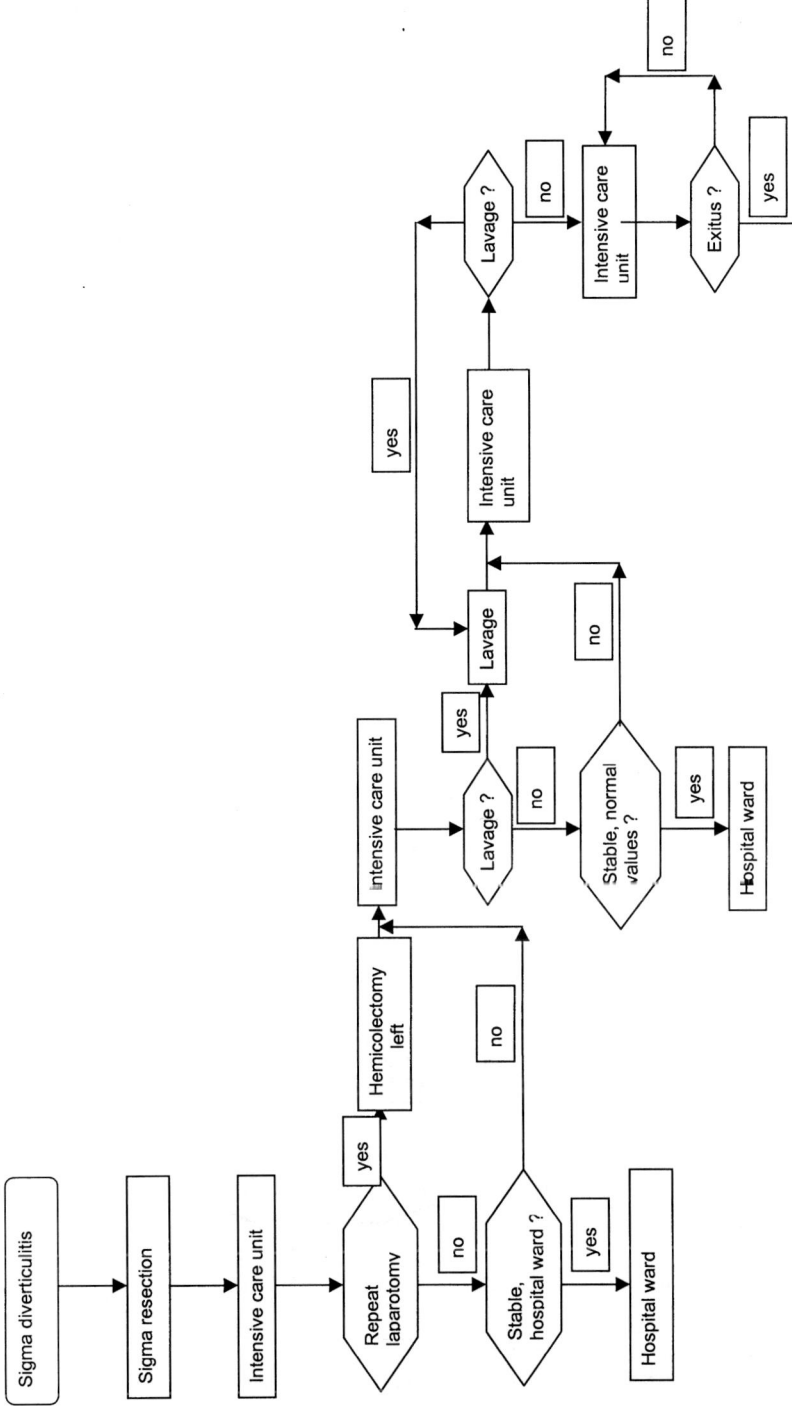

Fig. 11. Algorithm of a sigma diverticulitis patient with medical complications

the so-called CASA-Scores (Clinical Algorithm Structural Analysis-Score) were calculated by the ALGO v. 5.1 program.

Formula for the calculation of CASA-Sores:

CASA =   2 × number of Decision-Boxes.
            + number of all Action- and Clinical-State-Boxes (only the first in a line of Action- and Clinical-State-Boxes is counted).
            + the sum of all loops in the algorithm (equals the number of boxes between the origin and the re-entry of the loop into the algorithm, this requires that only boxes that can occur more than once are counted).

In that way, different elements of the algorithm are weighted and can therefore be summed. Therefore, the CASA-Scores compare the structural complexity of clinical algorithms, independent of their content (Pearson et al. 1992).

The average mortality for patients with septic shock was 46.4% (see also table 18). Hemofiltration was medically indicated in 59.3% of cases, 60.5% of the patients were male and had an average CASA-Score of 31.7. The mortality rate of 61.3% amongst patients over 60 was significantly higher than that of 37.7% in the under 60 age group. An indication of hemofiltration also indicated a bad prognosis (69.7% mortality) whilst the control group only exhibited a mortality rate of 31.4%. With respect to the CASA-Score, there was a significant difference between younger patients (<60 years), which had an average score of 34.3 compared to 27.6 for older patients ≥60 years. There were no significant differences in the CASA-Scores between the sexes, between patients receiving, or not, hemofiltration, or between dead patients and survivors.

Surviving patients (<60 years) had an average CASA-Score of 38.3, whilst deceased patients had an average score of 27.2 ($p < 0.05$). The group containing patients ≥60 years old exhibited a reversed ratio (CASA-Score of survivors: 21.6; CASA-Score of deceased patients: 31.4). The difference in the patient group (<60

Table 18. Patients study variables and CASA-Score; Data are shown as mean ± SD

Group	n	CASA-Score	Age	Mortality (%)	Dialyses (%)
All patients	84	31.7±26.9	54.6±15.1	46.4	59.3
Deceased patients	39	29.3±23.1	58.0±16.2	100	59.0
Survivors	45	33.9±29.6	51.8±13.4	0	22.2
Male	52	31.8±26.9	55.0±14.0	52.8	44.2
Female	32	36.±29.9	54.0±16.6	34.4	31.3
Hemofiltration (indicated) patients	50	35.0±25.8	53.5±15.8	69.7	100
Non-hemofiltration patients	34	29.7±27.4	55.3±14.6	31.4	0
≥ 60 years	31	27.6±19.0	69.5±5.2	61.3	38.7
< 60 years	53	34.3±30.4	45.8±11.7	37.7	39.6

years) was found to be statistically significant, this significance could not be demonstrated in the ≥ 60 year patient group.

There was no significant difference in the hemofiltration-indicated group when comparing the CASA-Score and mortality. Nevertheless, the survivors of the non-hemofiltration group had a significantly higher CASA-Score of 34.4 compared to that of 19.5 ($p < 0.05$) in the deceased group.

The basis of this study was the fact that the heterogeneity of treatment can be quantified by the utilization of clinical algorithms. The literature provides several examples where clinical algorithms prove to be a valid method for the demonstration not only of structural but also qualitative differences in therapy management. This has been shown by Pearson, Margolis and others for two different diseases/therapies (nodular change in the thyroid gland and sinusitis) (Pearson et al. 1992). As there is no "golden standard" for the measurement the structural complexity of algorithms, the CASA-Score derived values were compared with the estimations of 56 clinicians, who were asked to select one of six blank algorithms offered to them. CASA values and those derived by clinical experience were shown to demonstrate a high concordance. As no better method than the use of clinical experience for the judging of the complexity of clinical treatment is known, it therefore has to be concluded that CASA is a valid method (Sitter et al.; Pearson et al. 1992).

The present study has facilitated the use of the experience gained with CASA-Scores, to compare, independent of context, the structural differences of clinical algorithms. It has also be shown at the conference of the Lucerne Sepsis Study Group in Marburg, Germany, that models for measuring the heterogeneity of therapy management are indeed able to demonstrate differences in case related management. Here, 22 centers have centrally developed an algorithm, based on a single case causal model (70 year old patient with colorectal-carcinoma and a post-operative anastomoses insufficiency). The CASA-Scores were found to vary between 20 and 168, demonstrating a wide variation in the heterogeneity of therapy (Encke et al. 1997). The fact that differences in the complexity are also reflected by the outcome has also been shown in the present study. Although there was no significant difference in the CASA-Scores between survivors and diseased patients, a significantly higher value was demonstrated for the survivors (38.3) in the < 60 years group compared to the deceased group (27.2). This is a surprising finding, as intuition would suggest the opposite result. To draw the conclusion that the low therapy-complexity is directly responsible for the non-survival, is in our view not valid; a prospective study would be necessary in order to conclude what is cause and effect.

There are only few accepted general rules for the therapy of abdominal sepsis and consequently for septic shock. One of these is the sanitation of the infectious site by surgical means (Berger and Buttenschoen 1998; Christou et al. 1993; Hau et al. 1995). A wide range of studies, examining the therapy of abdominal peritonitis using different techniques, do not demonstrate a significant difference in the mortality rate between techniques (Berger and Buttenschoen 1998), however, the comparability of these studies is limited. The increase in mortality, related to the number of repeat-laparotomies (35.7% mortality after a single repeat-laparotomy, 50% with two and 70% with more than two) as described by

Koperna and Schulz (Koperna and Schulz 1996) could not be confirmed in our study. This is due to the similar CASA-Scores between the survivor and deceased patient groups.

Patients that were younger than 60 years and patients with a medical indication for hemofiltration do indeed benefit from repeat laparotomies, irrespective of whether the laparotomy was by patient demand or part of the therapy plan. This improving effect could not be seen in patients ≥ 60 years of age.

In this study, a great deal of experience was gained in the application of clinical algorithms. These are useful tools for the comparison of different therapy regimes, even though their practical application can be problematic; this is particularly true for their use in multi-center studies. A major source of problems is the design of the algorithm, where small deviations can cause huge differences in the CASA-Score. Therefore, it is required that the multi-center studies centralize their development of algorithms. However, this does not guarantee that the algorithms will not show a great heterogeneity, but the difference is that the heterogeneity is no longer due to structural differences; in fact differences in the treatment of the syndromes will be the main reason for the heterogeneity. Therefore, algorithms provide a potentially valid method for the description of the structural complexity of clinical attendance (Pearson et al. 1992). This will not solve the problem of heterogeneity in patient groups for future sepsis studies, but at least makes it possible to quantify the problem. Finally, it is evident from the study, controlling heterogeneity of sepsis trials is an illusion.

4.5.2
Computer Based Decision Support System in Septic Shock (www.medan.de)

Different scoring systems have been developed not only in order to document progression but also to estimate prognosis in the early treatment of sepsis. The systems to be mentioned are the APACHE-II-System ("acute physiology and chronic health evaluation system II") (Knaus et al. 1985), the MOF-Score (Goris et al. 1985), the "Sepsis-score of Elebute and Stoner" (Grundmann et al. 1988), the "Mannheim-Peritonitis-Index" (MPI) (Wacha et al. 1987) and the "injury severity score" (ISS) (Baker et al. 1974).

The present problem, which is to evaluate a course with different patient variables and to predict future progression, corresponds to the general problem of time series analysis (Brause 1995).

An important, methodically relevant area that uses serial kinetic analysis is for instance in the prediction of share and exchange rates, with the help of different variables such as the share index, the dollar exchange rate and other economical indices. In contrast to conventional methods such as the Fourrier-analysis or gliding mean values, their success is based on the utilisation of adaptable systems, namely artificial neuronal networks. For this, the network is trained with known data until it not only correctly predicts the known events from the past but also achieves sufficient precision with new data.

The networks used for this can also be called approximation-networks since they are asked to give the best possible approximation for a corresponding value of an unknown function with a given set of parameters.

Neuronal networks are also called "artificial neuronal networks"; they are information-transforming systems consisting of a huge number of simple "cells" that send information to each other by the activation of cells via directed connections (analogous to the action potentials of "real" neurons).

The basic elements or neurons are (in general) organised in layers. Every neuron is connected to those in the subsequent layers. Distinct networks differ in their utilisation in different aspects, but certain properties can be found in all neuronal networks in use today:

- neural networks "learn" by experience;
- they are particularly useful in areas, where conventional statistics fail, such as when dealing with complex and non-linear problems;
- the number of cases necessary in order to obtain optimal results depends on the type of problem and the number of initial variables.

Today's most common types of neuronal networks are the "multi-layer perceptron", the "radial-base-function" and the Kohonen-network. For the purposes of our analysis, we used the first two, namely the "multilayer-perceptron" and the "radial-base-function" networks.

As already mentioned, neuronal networks are particularly adapted to solve complex, non-linear problems. Whereas in conventional statistics the requirements of the analysed data are very high (there has to be a linear correlation and the random samples have to meet normal distribution, something which is rarely found in medicine) the neuronal networks are essentially less pretentious, such that with the exception of the data being representative, there is hardly any other requirement.

In contrast to neuronal networks, scoring systems are often used in intensive care medicine (Foitzik et al. 1995; Ohmann and Groos-Weege 1992; Wahl et al 1996). The scoring systems currently used to predict the survival of patients in intensive care units are highly specific, meaning that they predict the survival in about 90% of all cases, but they are not very sensitive, meaning that they only predict death in $50\pm70\%$ of all cases. For this reason it is generally recommended that these scoring systems should only be used for groups of patients, and not for individuals (Suter et al. 1994). In common with each other, the scoring systems mentioned use variables that are all handled as independent events. This can lead to a significant loss of precious information with predictive value. By the use of logistic regression it was attempted to take this critical point into consideration, however it has to be stated that the very complex situation of intensive care patients cannot be recorded by this means. Neuronal networks have proven especially useful for such applications since they can reflect the "chaotic behaviour" of biological processes (Baxt 1994).

Nowadays, neuronal networks are used in different clinical areas: for appendicitis (Eberhard et al. 1991) and heart attack (Baxt 1991), in the analysis of EEG and ECG information (Bortolan and Willems 1993; Clayton et al. 1994; Devine and Macfarlane 1993; Edenbrandt et al. 1993; Kloppel 1994; Masic and Pfurtscheller 1993), as well as liver transplantation (Doyle et al. 1994) and cardiac valve surgery (Katz et al. 1993).

A recently published study for intensive care medicine compared the performance of a neuronal network with a logistic regression model for patients with septic shock (Dybowski et al. 1996); the neuronal network exhibited much better results. However, one aspect of this study is worth criticising, namely that a single day of the intensive care period was randomly chosen without the date being specified. In reality this means that the initial as well as the final dates of the intensive care period have been used in this study. Therefore this neuronal network is useless in a clinical situation. A neuronal network is required at the beginning of the period of critical development. This requirement is only met when the parameters of the 1st day or changes from the 1st to the 2nd day of patients with septic shock are introduced into the neuronal network. Then, sensitivity and specificity reaches almost 100% and this in view there is a failure of the APACHE II score, which is found to be identical for surviving and deceased patients with septic shock (Hanisch et al. 1998). The neuronal network should be further developed by including the observations of the dynamics of septic progression. This could enable an individual prognosis with the aim of indicating the danger of a lethal progression as early as possible and to counteract this development by all possible means.

Finally we would like to underline the fact that information through neuronal networks constitutes a level of support, which does not restrict the practitioner. Under no circumstances do we interpret the use of neuronal networks in a fatalistic way as is currently being done with a prognostic system (headline "death computer"). Naturally the use of a "machine" giving information about life and death is highly emotive; however, we assume that once databases extend to several centres and thus the heterogeneity of the clinical features is adequately considered, it will be possible to establish, very early on, any alarm signals that might allow timely treatment and thus the lowering of the world-wide rates of mortality due to septic shock, which are still very high. In this context we would like to cite the philosopher Churchland: "... artificial neuronal networks will soon enable diagnosis which will be more reliable, faster and more logical than man could ever be. Such networks will also be capable of establishing proposals for treatment in a faster and more judicious way than any practitioner"[Churchland 1997). The project medan has been launched in this direction (www.medan.de).

References

American College of Chest Physicans/Society of Critical Care Medicine Consensus Conference: Definitions for sepsis and organ failure and guidelines for the use of innovative therapies in sepsis. Crit Care Med 20: 864–874

Apte NM, Karnad DR, Medhekar TP, Tilve GH, Morye S, Bhave GG (1992) Gastric colonization and pneumonia in intubated critical ill patients receiving stress ulcer prophylaxis: A randomized, controlled trial. Crit Care Med 20: 590–593

Artigas A, Bernard G, Carlet J, Dreyfuss D, Gattioni L, Hudson L, Lamy M, Marini J, Matthay M, Pinsky M, Spragg R, Suter P and the Consensus Committee: (1998) The American-European Consensus Conference on ARDS, Part 2: Ventilatory, Pharmacologic, Supportive Therapy,

Study Design Strategies, and Issues Related to Recovery and Remodeling. Am J Respir Crit Care Med 157: 1332–1347

Baker SP, O'Neill B, Haddon W, Long WB (1974) The injury severity score: A method for describing patients with multiple injuries and evaluation emergency care. J Trauma 14: 187

Banks JG, Foulis AK, Ledingham IMcA, MacSween RNM (1982) Liver function in septic shock. J Clin Pathol 35: 1249

Bastos P, Xiaolu S, Wagnder DP, Wu A et al. (1993) Glasgow Coma Scale score in the evaluation of outcome in the intensive care unit: findings from the Acute Physiology and Chronic Health Evaluation III study. Crit Care Med 21: 1459

Baxt WG (1991) Use of an artificial neural network for the diagnosis of myocardial infarction. Ann Intern Med 115: 843

Baxt WG (1994) Complexity, chaos and human physiology: the justification for non-linear neural computational analysis. Cancer Let 77: 85

Becker SD, Lamont JT (1988) Postoperative jaundice. Semin Liver Dis 8: 183

Bein Th, Fröhlich D, Frey A, Metz Ch et al. (1995) Vergleich von APACHE-II und APACHE-III zur Einschätzung der Erkrankungsschwere von Intensivpatienten. Anaesthesist 44: 37

Ben-Menachem T, Fogel R, Patel RV, Touchette M, Zarowitz B, Hadzijahic N, Divine G, Verter I, Bresalier R (1994) Prophylaxis for stress-related gastric hemorrhage in the medical intensive care unit. Ann Int Med 121: 568–575

Berger D, Beger HG (1991) Neue Aspekte zur Pathogenese und Behandlung der Sepsis und des septischen Schocks. Chirurg 62: 783–788

Berger D, Buttenschoen K (1998) Management of abdominal sepsis. Langenbeck's Arch Surg 383: 35–43

Bernard G, Artigas, Brigham K, Carlet J, Falke K, Hudson L, Lamy, Legall J, Morris A, Spragg R and the Consensus Committee (1994) The American-European Consensus Conference on ARDS-Definitions, Mechanism, Relevant Outcomes, and Clinical Trial Coordination. Am J Respir Crit Care Med 149: 818–824

Betzler M (1998) Chirurgisch-technische Leitlinien bei intestinaler Ischämie. Chirurg 69: 1–7

Boley SJ, Kaley RN, Brandt LJ (1992) Mesenteric venous thrombosis. Surg Clin North Am 72: 183–201

Bone RC (1991) Let's agree on terminology: Definitions of sepsis. Crit Care Med 19: 973–976

Bone RC (1991) Sepsis, the sepsis syndrome, multi organ failure: A plea for comparable definitions. Ann Intern Med 14: 332–333

Bone RC (1991) The pathogenesis of sepsis. Ann Intern Med 115: 457–469

Bone RC (1994) Sepsis and its complications: The clinical problem. Crit Care Med 22: S8–11

Bone RC (1996) Why sepsis trials fail. JAMA 276: 565–566

Bone RC, Balk RA, Cerra FB, Dellinger RP, Fein AM, Knaus WA, Schein RM, Sibbald WJ (1992)

Bortolan G, Willems JL (1993) Diagnostic ECG classification based on neural networks. J Electrocardiol 26: 75

Brandt LJ, Boley SJ (1992) Colonic ischemia. Surg Clin North Am 72: 203–229

Brause R (1995) Neuronale Netze. Teubner, Stuttgart

Brooks GS, Zimbler AG, Bodenheimer HC Jr, Burckard KW (1991) Patterns of liver test abnormalities in patients with surgical sepsis. Am Surg 57: 656

Bruin-Buisson CB, Doyon F, Carlet J, Dellamonica P, Gonin F, Lepoutre A, Mercier JC, Offenstadt G, Regnier B (1995) Incidence, risk factors, and outcome of severe sepsis and septic shock in adults. JAMA 274: 968–974

Caricco CJ, Meakins JL, Marshall JC, Fry D, Maier RV (1986) Multiple-organ-failure syndrome. Arch Surg 121: 196

Caroli J, Paraf A, Champeau J, Desvignes M (1950) Les ictères des la gastrectomie. Arch Mal l'App Dig 39: 1057

Cheadle WG, Vitale GC, Mackie CR, Cuschieri A (1985) Prophylactic postoperative nasogastric decompression. Ann Surg 202: 361–366

Christou NV, Barie PS, Dellinger EP, Waymack JP, Stone HH (1993) Surgical Infection Society intra-abdominal infection study. Prospective evaluation of management techniques and outcome. Arch Surg 128: 193–198

Chu CM, Chang CH, Liang YF (1987) Jaundice following open heart surgery. Ann Surg 165: 217

Churchland P (1997) Die Seelenmaschine. Spektrum, Heidelberg

Clarke RSJ, Doggart JR, Lavery T (1976) Changes in liver function after different types of surgery. Br J Anaesth 48: 119

Clayton RH, Murray A, Campbell RW (1994) Recognition of ventricular fibrillation using neural networks. Med Biol Eng Comput 32: 217

Cook DJ, Fuller HD, Guyatt GH, Marshall JC, Leasa D, Hall R, Winton TL, Rutledge F, Todd TJR, Roy P, Lacroix J, Griffith L, Willan A (1994) Risk factors for gastrointestinal bleeding in critically ill patients. N Engl J. Med 330: 377–381

Cook DJ, Laine LA, Guyatt GH, Raffin ThA (1991) Nosocomial pneumonia and the role of gastric pH. A metaanalysis. Chest 11: 7–13

Cook DJ, Reeve BK, Guyatt GH, Heyland DK, Griffith LE, Buckingham L, Tryba M (1996) Stress ulcer prophylaxis in critically ill patients. JAMA 275: 308–314

Current trends increase in national hospital discharge survey rates for septicemia – United States, 1979 – 1987. (1990) MMWR 39: 31–34

Daschner F, Reuschenbach K, Pfisterer I, Kappstein I, Vogel W, Krieg N, Just H (1987) Der Einfluß von Streßulkusprophylaxe auf die Häufigkeit einer Beatmungspneumonie. Anaesthesist 36: 9–18

Devine B, Macfarlane PW (1993) Detection of electrocardiographic "left ventricular strain" using neural nets. Med Biol Eng Comput 31: 343

Doberneck RC (1991) Revision and closure of the colostomy. Surg Clin North Am 71: 193–201

Doyle HR, Dvorschik I, Mitchell S, Marino S et al. (1994) Predicting outcome after liver transplantation: a connectionist approach. Ann Surg 219: 408

Driks MR, Craven DE, Celli BR, Manning M, Burke RA, Garvin GM, Kunches LM, Farber HW, Wedel SA, McCabe WR (1987) Nosocomial pneumonia in intubated patients given sucralfate as compared with antacids or histamine type 2 blockers. N Eng J Med 317: 1376-1382

Dybowski R, Weller P, Chang R, Grant V (1996) Prediction of outcome in critically ill patients using artificial neural networks synthesised by genetic algorithm. Lancet 347: 1146

Eberhard RC, Dobbins RW, Hutton LV (1991) Neural Network paradigm comparisons for appendicitis diagnosis. Proceedings of the fourth annual IEEE Symposium on Computer-based Medical Systems, p 298

Edenbrandt L, Heden B, Pahlm O (1993) Neural networks for analysis of ECG complexes. J Electrocardiol 26: 74

Elebute EA, Stoner HB (1983) The grading of sepsis. Br J Surg 70: 29

Encke A, Hanisch E, Sitter H, Greger B, Bauhofer A, Margolis C et al. (1997) Evaluation models for therapy planning/standardization exemplified by infection. Langenbeck's Arch Chir Suppl Kongressband 114: 323–329

Eypasch E, Troidl H, Mennigen R, Spangenberger W, Barlow A (1992) Laparoscopy via an indwelling cannula: an alternative to planned relaparotomy. Br J Surg 79: 1395

Ferraris VA (1983) Exploratory laparotomy for potential abdominal sepsis in patients with multiple organ failure. Arch Surg 118: 1130–1133

Foitzik Th, Holle R, Schall R, Moesta Th et al. (1995) Der Heidelberger Wachstation-Score. Chirurg 66: 513

Franson TR, LaBrecque DR, Buggy BP, Harris GJ, Hoffmann RG (1989) Serial bilirubin determinations as a prognostic marker in clinical infection. Am J Med Sci 296: 149

Goris RJA (1989) Multiple organ failure: whole body inflammation. Schweiz Med Wochenschr 119: 347

Goris RJA, Boekholtz WKF, van Bebber IPT, Nuytinck JKS, Schillings PHM (1986) Multiple-organ failure and sepsis without bacteremia. Arch Surg 121: 897

Goris RJA, te Boekhorst TPA, Nuytinck JKS, Gimrere JSF (1985) Multiple organ failure ± generalized autodestructive inflammation? Arch Surg 120: 1109

Grundmann R, Kipping N, Wesoly C (1988) Der "Sepsisscore" von Elebute und Stoner zur Definition der postoperativen Sepsis auf der Intensivstation. Intensivmedizin 25: 268

Guthrie LG (1903) On the fatal effects of chloroform on children suffering from a peculiar condition of fatty liver. Lancet 2: 10

Hanisch E, Büssow M, Brause R, Encke A (1998) Individuelle Prognose bei kritisch kranken Patienten mit septischem Schock durch ein neuronales Netz?Chirurg 69: 77–81

Hanley J, McNeil B (1982) The meaning and use of the area under a Receiver Operating Caracteristic (ROC) Curve Radiology 143: 29

Hartmann H (1921) Nouveau procède d'ablation des cancers de la partie terminale du colon pelvier. Congrès Francais de Chirurgie 30: 411–418

Hau T, Ohmann C, Wohnershauser A, Wache H, Yang Q (1995) Planned relaparotomy vs relaparotomy on demand in the treatment of intraabdominal infections. The Peritonitis Study Group of the Surgical Infection Society Europe. Arch Surg 130: 1193–1196

Hau T, Ohmann C, Wolmershäuser A, Wacha H, Yang Q for the Peritonitis Study Group of the Surgical Infection Society-Europe (1995) Planned relaparotomy vs relaparotomy on demand in the treatment of intraabdominal infections. Arch Surg 130: 1193–1197

Hawker F (1991) Liver dysfunction in critical illness. Anaesth Intesive Care 19: 165

Hawley PR (1973) Causes and prevention of colonic anastomotic breakdown. Dis Colon Rectum 16: 272–277

Herbrecht PJ, Garrison N, Fry DE (1984) Early urgent relaparotomy. Arch Surg 119: 369–374

Herfarth Ch, Körner K (1965) Beitrag zum Problem des postoperativen Ikterus. Chirurg 36: 313

Irvin TT, Goligher JC (1970) Aetiology and disruption of intestinal anastomoses. Br J Surg 119: 1–8

Kaleya R, Sammartano B, Boley S (1992) Aggressive approach to acute mesenteric ischemia. Surg Clin North Am 72: 157–173

Karlstadt RG, Iberti TJ, Siverstein J, Lindenberg L, Bright-Asare P, Rockhold F, Young MD (1990) Comparison of cimetidine and placebo for the prophylaxis of upper gastrointestinal bleeding due to stress-related gastric mucosal damage in the intensive care unit. J Intensive Care Med 5: 26–32

Katz AS, Katz S, Wickham E, Quijano RC et al. (1993) Prediction of valve-related complications for artificial heart valves using adaptive neural networks: a preliminary study. J Heart Valve Dis 2: 504

Khoury DA, Beck DR, Opelka FG, Hicks TC, Timmcke AE, Gathright JB Jr (1996) Colostomy closure: Ochsner clinic experience. Dis Colon Rectum 39: 605–609

Kloppel B (1994) Application of neural networks for EEG analysis. Consideration and first results. Neuropsychobiology 29: 39

Knaus WA (1988) The science of prediction and its implications for the clinician today. Theor Surg 3: 93

Knaus WA, Draper EA, Wagner DP, Zimmermann JE (1985) APACHE II: A severiy of disease classification system. Crit Care Med 13: 818

Knaus WA, Draper EA, Wagner DP, Zimmermann JE (1985) Prognosis in acute organ-system failure. Ann Surg 202: 685

Koperna T, Schulz F (1996) Prognosis and treatment of peritonitis. Do we need new scoring systems? Arch Surg 131: 180–186

Koruth NM, Krukowski ZH, Youngson GG et al. (1985) Intraoperative colonic irrigation in the management of left-sided large bowel emergencies. Br J Surg 72: 708–711

Krenzien I, Lorenz W (1990) Scoring-Systeme für schwere intraabdominelle Infektionen. Zentralbl Chir 115: 1065

MacSweeney S, Postelthwaite J (1994) "Second look" laparoscopy in the management of acute mesenteric ischemia. Br J Surg 81: 90

Maier RV, Mitchell D, Gentilello L (1994) Optimal therapy for stress gastritis. Ann Surg 220: 353–363

Marshal JC (2000) Clinical trials of mediator-directed therapy in sepsis: what have we learned? Intensive Care Med 26: 75–83

Marshall J, Sweeney D (1990) Microbial infection and the septic response in critical surgical illness: sepsis, not infection, determines outcome. Arch Surg 125: 17–23

Marshall, JC, Cook, DJ, Christou, NV, Bernard, GR et al. (1995) Multiple Organ Dysfunction Score: A reliable descriptor of a complex clinical outcome Crit Care Med 23: 1638

Martin C, Leone M, Ayem M-L (2000) How to use norepinephrine in septic shock patients. Intensivmed 37: 507–513

Martin LF, Booth F, Karlstadt RG, Silverstein JH, Jacobs DM, Hampsey I, Bowman SC, D'Ambrosio CA (1993) Continuous intravenous cimetidine decreases stress-related upper gastrointestinal hemorrhage without promoting pneumonia. Crit Care Med 21: 19–30

Masic N, Pfurtscheller G (1993) Neural network based classification of single trial EEG data. Artif Intell Med 5: 503

Metz CA, Livingston DH, Smith Ist, Larson GM, Wilson TH (1993) Impact of multiple risk factors and ranitidine prophylaxis on the development of stress-related upper gastrointestinal bleeding: a prospective, multicenter, double-blind, randomized trial. Crit Care Med 21: 1844-1849

Miller DJ, Keeton GR, Webber GR, Saunder SJ (1976) Jaundice in severe bacterial infection. Gastroenterology 71: 94

Mitsudo S, Brandt L (1992) Pathology of intestinal ischemia. Surg Clin North Am 72: 43–63

Murray B, Fakhry SM, Cooney R, Rutledge R, Meyer AA (1992) Comparison of ICU nursis clinical judgement and APACHE II score in predicting ICU outcome in critical ill surgical patients. Crit Care Med 20: 57

Nel CJ, Pretorius DJ, de Vaal JB (1986) Reoperating for suspected intraabdominal sepsis in the critically ill patients. S Afr J Surg 24: 60–62

O'Higging NJ (1989) Effect of mechanical bowel preparation on anastomotic integrity following low anterior resection on dogs. Br J Surg 76: 756–758

Ohmann C, Grofs-Weege W (1992) Scoring-Systeme auf der chirurgischen Intensivstation. Chirurg 63: 1021

Ohmann C, Groß-Weege W (1992) Scoring-Systeme auf der chirurgischen Intensivstation Chirurg 63: 1021

Parrillo JE (1993) Pathogenetic mechanism of septic shock. N Engl J Med 328: 1471–1477

Pearson SD, Margolis CZ, Davis S, Schreier LK, Gottlieb LK (1992) The clinical algorithm nosology: A method for comparing algorithmic guidelines. Med Decis Making 12: 123–131

Pickworth KK, Falcone RE, Hoogeboom JE, Santanello SA (1993) Occurrence of nosocomial pneumonia in mechanically ventilated trauma patients. Crit Care Med 12: 1856–1862

Pitcher WD, Musher DM (1982) Critical importance of early diagnosis and treatment of intraabdominal infection. Arch Surg 117: 328–333

Pittet D, Rangel-Frausto S, Li N, Tarara D, Costigan M, Rempe L, Jebson P, Wenzel RP (1995) Systemic inflammatory response syndrome, sepsis, severe sepsis and septic shock: incidence, morbidities and outcome in surgical ICU patients. Intensive Care Med 21: 302–309

Polk HC, Jr, Shields CL (1977) Remote organ failure: a valid sign of occult intraabdominal infection. Surgery 81: 310–313

Prod'hom G, Leuenberger P, Koerfer J, Blum A, Chiolero R, Schaller MD, Perret C, Spinnler O, Blondel J, Siegrist H, Saghafi L, Blanc D, Francioli P (1994) Nosocomial pneumonia in mechanically ventilated patients receiving antacid. Ann Intern Med 120: 653–662

Proposal for clinical algorithm standards. Society for Medical Decision Making. Committee on Standardization of Clinical Algorithms. Med Decis Making 1992; 12: 149–154

Pulmonary Artery Catheter Consensus Conference (1997) Consensus statement. Crit Care Med 25: 910–925

Pusajó JF, Bumaschny E, Doglio GR, Cherjovsky M, Lipinszki AI, Hernández MS, Egurrola MA (1993) Postoperative intraabdominal sepsis requiring reoperation – value of a predictive index. Arch Surg 128: 218–223

Rangel-Frausto S, Pittet D, Costigan M, Hwang T, Davis CS, Wenzel RP (1995) The natural history of the systemic inflammatory response syndrome (SIRS). JAMA 273: 117–123

Reusser P, Zimmerli W, Scheidegger D, Marbet GA, Buser M, Gyr K (1989) Role of gastric colonization in nosocomial infections and endotoxemia: A prospective study in neurosurgical patients. J Infect Dis 160: 414–421

Rixen D, Siegel JH, Friedman HP (1996) "Sepsis/SIRS," Physiologic classification, severity stratification, relation to cytokine elaboration and outcome prediction in posttrauma critical illness. J Trauma 41: 581

Ronco C, Bellomo R, Homel P, Brendolan A, Dan M, Piccini P, La Greca G (2000) Effects of different doses in continuous venovenous haemofiltration on outcomes of acute renal failure: a prospective randomised trial. Lancet 355: 26–30

Sackier J (1992) Diagnostic laparoscopy in nonmalignant disease. Surg Clin North Am 72: 1033–1043

Salvo I, De Cian W, Musicco M, Langer M, Piandena R, Wolfler A, Montani C, Magni E (1995) The Italian sepsis study: preliminary results on the incidence and evolution of SIRS, sepsis severe sepsis and septic shock. Intensive Care Med 21: 244–249

Schein M, Wittmann DH, Wise L, Condon RE (1997) Abdominal contamination, infection and sepsis: a continuum. Br J Surg 84: 269–272

Schmid M, Hefti ML, Gattiker R (1965) Benign postoperative intrahepatic cholestasis. N Engl J Med 272: 545

Schneider TA, Longo WE, Ure T, Vernava AM, III (1994) Mesenteric ischemia. Acute arterial syndromes. Dis Colon Rectum 37: 1163–1174

Schottmüller H (1914) Wesen und Behandlung der Sepsis. Inn Med 31: 257

Schriefers KH, Wenn B (1967) Über den Ikterus nach operativen Eingriffen. Dtsch Med Wochenschr 92: 540

Schuster DP (1993) Stress ulcer prophylaxis: In whom? With what? Crit Care Med 21: 4–6

Seekamp A, Regel G, Sturm JA, Tscherne H (1991) Das Leberversagen als Teil eines Multiorganversagens nach Polytrauma. Unfallchirurg 94: 502

Short A, Cumming A (1999) ABC of intensive care. Renal support. BMJ 319: 41–43

Sibbald WJ, Doig G, Inman KJ (1995) Sepsis, SIRS and infection. Intensive Care Med 21: 299–301

Sibbald WJ, Marshall J, Christou N, Girotti M, Mc Cormack D, Rostein O, Martin C, Meakins J (1991) "Sepsis"-Clarity of existing terminology or more confusion? Crit Care Med 19: 996–998

Sinanan M, Maier RV, Carrico CJ (1984) Laparotomy for intraabdominal sepsis in patients in an intensive care unit. Arch Surg 119: 652–658

Sitter H, Dietz W, Stinner B, Geks I, Bauhofer A, Celik I et al. (1999) Clinical guidelines as part of total quality management. Analysis of heterogenous treatment concepts of sepsis in various clinics with computer assisted generation, logical testing and complexity assessment of clinical algorithms. Zentralbl Chir 124: 318–326

Slutzki S, Halpern Z, Negri M, Kais H, Halevy A (1996) The laparoscopic second look for ischemic bowel disease. Surg Endosc 10: 729–731

Smith SRG, Connolly JC, Gilmore OJA (1983) The effect of faecal loading on colonic anastomotic healing. Br J Surg 70: 49–50

Sprung CL (1991) Definitions of sepsis-Have we reached a consensus? Crit Care Med 19: 849–851

Sugrue M (2000) Intraabdominal pressure and intensive care: current concepts and future implications. Intensivmed 37: 529–535

Suter P, Armaganidis A, Beaufils F, Bonfill X et al. (1994) Predicting outcome in ICU patients. Intensive Care Med 20: 390

Task Force of the American College of Critical Care Medicine, Society of Critical Care Medicine (1999) Practice parameters for hemodynamic support of sepsis in adult patients in sepsis. Crit Care Med 27: 639–660

te Brekhorst Th, Urlus M, Doesburg W, Yap SH, Goris RJA (1988) Etiologic factors of jaundice in severly ill patients. J Hepatol 7: 111

Tilney NL, Bailey GL, Morgan AP (1973) Sequential system failure after rupture of abdominal aortic aneurysms: An unsolved problem in postoperative care. Ann Surg 108: 117

Tryba M, Zevounou F, Wruck G (1988) Streßblutungen und postoperative Pneumonien bei Intensivpatienten unter Ranitidin oder Pirenzepin. Dtsch Med Wschr 113: 930–936

Tryba M (1988) Prevention of stress bleeding with ranitidine or pirenzipine and the risk of pneumonia. J Clin Anaesth1: 12–20

Tryba M (1989) Side effects of stress bleeding prophylaxis. Am J Med 86 (Suppl 6A): 85–93

van Goor H (1997) Surgical treatment of severe intraabdominal infection. Hepatogastroenterology 44: 975–981

Vincent JL (1997) Dear SIRS, I'm sorry to say I don't like you... Crit Care Med 25: 372–374

Vincent J-L, De Mendonca A, Cantraine F, Moreno et al. (1998) Use of the SOFA score to assess the incidence of organ dysfunction/failure in intensive care units: Results of a multicenter, prospective study. Crit Care Med (1998) 26: 1793

Vincent J-L, Moreno R, Takala J, Willatts S et al. (1996) The SOFA (Sepsis-related Organ Failure Assessment) score to describe organ dysfunction/failure. Intensive Care Med 22: 707

Wacha H, Lindner MM, Feldmann U, Wesch G et al. (1987) Mannheim peritonitis index ± prediction of risk of death from peritonitis: Construction of a statistical and validation of an empirically based index. Theor Surg 1: 169

Wahl W, Pelletier K, Schmidtmann S, Junginger Th (1996) Erfahrungen mit verschiedenen Scores zur Beurteilung der Prognose bei postoperativen Intensivtherapiepatienten. Chirurg 67: 710

Winkeltau GJ, Bertram P, Braun J, Schumpelick V (1996) Die differenzierte chirurgische Therapie der diffusen Peritonitis – eine prospektive Studie. Leber Magen Darm 26: 144–148

Zamir G, Reissman P (1998) Diagnostic laparoscopy in mesenteric ischemia. Surg Endosc 12: 390–393

Zandstra DF, Stoutenbeek CP (1994) The virtual absence of stress-ulceration related bleeding in ICU patients receiveing prolonged mechanical ventilation without any prophylaxis. A prospective cohort study. Intensive Care Med 20: 335–340

The Doctor's Dilemma: The Assessment of Successful Adjunctive Immunotherapy in Critically Ill Patients

H. G. KRESS

5.1
What is the Problem ... And Why Should It Be Solved?

Clinical trials are generally considered the most effective approach to evaluate the efficacy of any medical management, including the testing of therapeutic interventions. Their quality in design, execution and data analysis renders medicine more and more rational, scientifically sound and evidence-based. The results of clinical studies are essential in protecting patients from potential harm and the whole society from vasting the limited economic resources for questionable, ineffective or even harmful and costly treatments.

This is also true for the treatment of septic patients, and thus clinical trials must remain the gold standard for assessing efficacy and safety of new therapies of sepsis (Finch 1998). Besides enthusiasm, energy and organisational skills such trials demand a plausible hypothesis based on pre-clinical experimental data. In addition, the hypothesis to be tested should be consistent with the current understanding of the pathophysiology of the disease (Finch 1998).

Sepsis – and this term means the systemic response of the whole body to an infection – is an unresolved clinical problem. Epidemiologic data show that there is little evidence of substantial improvement in sepsis survival since the 1970s (Bone 1993). In the 1970s and 1980s the clinicians' and scientists' view was a rather simplistic one. The hope of finding a "magic bullet" to treat sepsis has been frustrating, and nowadays even fanatic optimists must have realised that no substance will represent such a magic agent that could dramatically improve the prognosis and outcome of sepsis.

During the last 30 years, more than 10000 patients have been enrolled in more than four dozens of randomised trials of "anti-sepsis" agents (Neugebauer et al. 1998). The progress in immunology, and molecular and cell biology has expanded our knowledge on systemic inflammatory response and the development of organ failure, and not only optimists have believed that it would be only a matter of time and more studies to solve the problem of sepsis and to find the breakthrough in its therapy. Although sound scientific reasons suggested the evaluation of these agents in human studies, based in most cases on supporting experimental evidence from animal models, all of the agents have produced more or less disappointing results from clinical trials. This therapeutic failure has been subject of a broad and ongoing scientific discussion on the methodology of previous studies and on future approaches to the complex problem of sepsis therapy. Antibiotics, anti-inflammatory (corticosteroids), adjunctive immunotherapeutic (polyclonal immunoglobulins), anti-endotoxin, and anti-mediator strategies (monoclonal antibodies, antagonists etc.) all failed to improve outcome as defined by the traditional primary endpoint of mortality. To be honest, also already established non-antiinfective, supportive therapies could not been shown to significantly improve mortality of these critically ill patients. For instance, catecholamines have never been investigated with respect to their impact on patient morbidity and mortality. Many diagnostic and therapeutic tools for critically ill patients have been introduced into clinical practice with insufficient evaluation of their impact on clinically important outcomes and their economic consequences (Sibbald and Vincent 1995 in Round table...). Fluid replacement, red blood cell transfusions and vasoactive drug therapy have been adopted in spite of a low-grade evidence from clinical studies (level II to V evidence using the "Levels of Evidence Grades of Recommendations" approach to assessing the clinical literature (Oxmann et al. 1993; Guyatt et al. 1994).

Nevertheless, we have now reached a point where traditional study designs for "anti-sepsis trials" should be re-evaluated in order to improve the methodology and – as a consequence – the quality and reliability of future trials on "anti-sepsis" treatments in critically ill patients. Based on the analysis of previous sepsis trials and their serious limitations and flaws, the purpose of this article is to suggest new criteria for the assessment of the therapeutic efficacy of immunotherapy and its impact on clinical outcome.

Interestingly enough, whereas international guidelines have been published and up-dated for the clinical evaluation of anti-infective drugs by a number of different authors and groups (Beam et al. 1992; Beam et al. 1993; Immunocompromised Host Society 1990), no guidelines exist for the evaluation of adjunctive immunotherapies. Thus, there is a considerable controversy on the design and conduct of trials in sepsis (Finch 1998; Sibbald and Vincent 1995 in Round table...), especially concerning such basic issues as the assessment of outcome with respect to both the definition of successful response or failure (Neugebauer et al. 1998). Within this context other crucial points are also to be addressed: Do current animal models actually reflect critical illness in ICU patients? Do we rely on evidence-based pathophysiological concepts of sepsis rather than on modern trendy (some people even would say "sexy") pathophysiological beliefs? May experimental data from animal models simply be (mis-)used for the design of therapeutic trials in humans (Piper et al. 1996) Is "anti-sepsis therapy" absolutely the same as "anti-infective" or "anti-inflammatory" strategies or has it a quality of its own? Is big always beautiful, e.g. are large multi-centre trials always superior to small, well-designed and closely monitored single-centre studies? No doubt, when we aim at wrong targets of treatment and study inappropriate endpoints, we will always obtain frustrating results (rubbish in – rubbish out).

5.2
Limitations, Pitfalls and Flaws of Trials on Adjunctive Immunotherapy

Although the clinical trial is the final arbiter of efficacy and safety in the treatment of critically ill patients, the history of therapeutic trials in sepsis has been one of unfulfilled expectations and conflicting results (Bone 1993; Neugebauer et al. 1998; Sibbald and Vincent 1995 in Round table...; Bone 1991; Warren et al. 1992). These trials have been conducted in intensive care units in a heterogeneous patient population with various entry criteria and endpoints of response. As outlined by Neugebauer et al. (1998), the major flaws have been the reliance on premature or inappropriate animal models, investigating heterogeneous patient populations under non-standardised intensive care regimens and ignoring pharmacokinetic and pharmacodynamic characteristics of the study drugs. One of the most serious flaws, however, was the choice of inappropriate endpoints for the assessment of successful treatment.

5.2.1
Definition of the Disease To Be Treated

The definition of the disease expression and the assessment of severity are essential for an accurate and reproducible evaluation of anti-infective or "anti-sepsis" treatment. An imprecise terminology used during the past 20 to 30 years led to confusion and difficulties in interpretation of comparative clinical investigations.

In sepsis studies, particular care must be taken to avoid mixing together different stages and expressions of sepsis, because there does not exist the "typical septic" patient. The term sepsis is not sufficient to describe the study population, and reliance on such terms alone is unlikely to assist in the evaluation of new therapeutic approaches. In contrast to animal studies, in clinical trials of sepsis, the definition of sepsis is descriptive, the term "sepsis" refers not to a disease but to a syndrome which is based on a categorical definition that relates only superficially to the pathophysiology of the condition, except for its emphasis on shock as an index of disease severity. The standardisation of terms such as "sepsis", "sepsis syndrome" (Bone et al. 1989), "septic shock" and "refractory septic shock" has been a significant advance and has been supplemented by the introduction of such terms as the "systemic inflammatory response" (SIRS) and "multiple organ dysfunction syndrome" (MODS) (Sibbald and Vincent 1995 in Round table...; Am. Coll. of Chest Physicians 1992; Bone et al. 1992; Marshall 1995). The broadness of the criteria on which diagnosis of sepsis is based, is illustrated by a recent study (Rangel-Frausto et al. 1995) that compiled the natural history of the systemic inflammatory response. In this study (Rangel-Fausto et al. 1995), the frequency rate of SIRS in three general intensive care units and three general wards in a tertiary healthcare institution was reported to be 68%. This high rate of SIRS established concern that the definition, although sensitive (i.e. most patients with the condition fulfil the criteria), is not specific (i.e. only few of those patients without the condition fulfil the criteria). These observations show that there is no "gold-standard" diagnostic test to identify patients with sepsis. Since the rationale for the use of adjunctive therapies in sepsis is based on a number of consumptions, the attention has focused on the nomenclature and clinical definition of sepsis used to select patients for therapeutic trials (Bone et al. 1989; Bone et al. 1992; Baumgartner et al. 1992; Knaus et al. 1985). This is particularly important as large multi-centre trials are needed to detect a significant effect of therapy. Therefore, more recently, these categorical definitions have been refined to acknowledge that it is not only infection but systemic inflammation that is the underlying disorder, hence the new term "systemic inflammatory response syndrome" (SIRS) and "severe sepsis" replace the former "septic syndrome". Although categorical definitions (i.e. SIRS, severe sepsis) may predict the risk of mortality, there is an extremely wide variation in survival rates from <10% to >90% (Marshall 1995) within each category. To improve the ability of clinical trials to determine the efficacy of novel adjunctive therapies for critical ill patients (Knaus et al. 1995), some investigators have suggested the classification of patients according to physiologic parameters of possible prognostic value (assuming these factors can me measured before treatment).

Nevertheless one has to keep in mind, that most ICU patients meet the SIRS criteria. Thus, there may be almost as many "SIRS" patients as there are "critically ill" patients. It is not warranted to lump together a large number of acutely ill patients with different disease states. Moreover, only three of four patients presenting with severe sepsis have documented infection (Brun-Buisson et al. 1995). Although patients with clinically suspected sepsis but without microbiological documentation and patients with documented infections share common risk factors and have a similar mortality risk, their response to adjunctive therapies may dramatically differ. Up to now we do not have a precise answer to this fundamental problem. Regardless of the definition chosen, however, it is now recognised that in all future for clinical trials these definitions should be combined with appropriate risk stratification or risk prediction methods.

5.2.2
Heterogeneity of Study Populations

Trials in critically ill patients present a unique challenge because the population studied is heterogeneous, sepsis often presents with various co-morbid disease states, and septic patients often receive different treatments for these co-morbid states that are dependent on study centre preferences. Patients presenting with sepsis range from a young, previously healthy individual with a sudden onset of urinary tract infection to a patient with cirrhosis suffering from multiple organ system failure, on prolonged ventilator support in an Intensive Care Unit following emergency surgery for a leaking abdominal aneurysm (Vincent 1995). Sepsis patients are complexly ill with multiple risk factors for short-term mortality.

The admission diagnosis and the underlying disease (e.g. cirrhosis) remain the major determinants of outcome (Gasche et al. 1995). Scoring systems primarily focus on the relative risk of death, whereas the degree of organ dysfunction and even quality of life are also important (Baumgartner et al. 1992; Knaus et al. 1985; Knaus et al. 1995). Scoring systems are influenced by therapeutic interventions, and although organ failure is an important determinant of outcome, it is not useful in defining the target population for adjunctive therapies, as patients with advanced organ failure may not benefit from any novel intervention. The predominant use of scoring system has the major problems of complexity and lack of pathophysiological basis (Vincent 1995). Because of our poor understanding of the pathophysiology of the different disease states, the criteria used to enter patients into interventional trials are crucial to permit to use the right treatment at the right time in the right group of patients. Therefore, it is important to consider the presence and the source of infection, the type of microorganism, the severity of the underlying disease, and the appropriateness of the non-trial study therapy. Especially mixing together septic patients with and without documented infections may obscure relevant therapeutic effects of the interventions tested. Therefore, the effects of therapy should be evaluated separately in infected and non-infected patients. As this distinction may not be evident at entry of the clinical trial, it may be re-evaluated retrospectively by a clinical evaluation committee.

As could be shown in septic patients (Rangel-Frausto et al. 1995), the frequency of positive blood cultures increases with increasing disease severity. Thus, bacteremia may play an important role in determining outcome of sepsis. Short-term mortality was modestly higher in patients with bacteremia even after controlling for severity of illness. But this increase in risk was only present during the first month, and most deaths occurred in patients with a rapidly fatal disease. Thus, a high percentage of patients with bacteremia will do well regardless of therapy, and a large group of those patients who do poorly have another rapidly fatal disease. In large clinical trials (Gasche et al. 1995), bacteremia was identified in less than 50% of patients with sepsis, and the admission demographic data (including physiologic variables modified by sepsis) did not allow reliable discrimination between bacteremic and non-bacteremic patients. However, the analysis of patients included in clinical trials only is somewhat biased by the exclusion criteria used to select the patient population, and may sometimes not reflect the real clinical setting. Nevertheless the incidence of shock development after admission was significantly higher in bacteremic patients included in such trials as a whole.

Furthermore, the influence of anti-microbial therapy on the prognosis of bacteremic and non-bacteremic sepsis has still to be defined. Early appropriate antibiotic treatment is associated with a 50% reduction in fatality rate compared to patients treated with antibiotics to which the infecting organisms were resistant (Kreger et al. 1980). Also other authors have identified the benefit of appropriate antibiotic therapy on the prognosis of bacteremic sepsis (Gasche et al. 1995). However, when bacteremia was complicated by clinically diagnosed shock or ARDS, infection mortality could not be lowered by initial adequate antibiotics or subsequent adequate therapy. In addition, anti-microbial treatment prior to the development of full sepsis has been recently identified as a risk factor for death (Gasche et al. 1995). In view of the importance of the micro-biological evaluation of patients for trials of sepsis, it is surprising that many of the published trials give very few details on the methods involved in documenting infection and on the crucial points mentioned above. The adequacy and timeliness of source control is an important determinant of outcome in severe infection, but an under-emphasised component of the design and evaluation of clinical trials in sepsis. It is striking that in most clinical trials of sepsis the surgical therapy has not been evaluated systematically in these patients, and that few, if any, include a manoeuvre directed towards the control of the source of infection in their design.

In conclusion, the confounding events in most of the sepsis trials performed so far include (Finch 1998): inappropriate anti-microbial therapy, inappropriate empirical therapy, inappropriate targeted therapy, delayed therapy, therapy of insufficient duration or insufficient dosage; inadequate medical or surgical management; underlying or unforeseen conditions such as pre-enrolment, undiagnosed fatal condition, major haemorrhage, post-enrolment fatal condition unrelated to sepsis; therapy withheld or withdrawn before outcome was clear. Although in randomised clinical trials, it must be assumed that these events and factors similarly influence the treatment and the placebo arms of the treatment, differences in management may represent a more significant variable if studies are so dispersed that they include only a few patients in each centre. Accordingly it is desirable for clinical trials to provide clear therapeutic protocols to standardise patient management as much as possible.

5.3
Single or Multi-centre Trials?

As large differences in medical education, clinical management concepts, treatment policies and financial restrictions can be assumed between various institutions in multi-centre trials, it is not surprising that the outcome will differ between ICUs. Two major issues arise in interpreting results of multi-centre mega-trials (Yusuf et al. 1984). First, the simplicity of the design imposes a reductionist model on any treatment effect – one size fits all. Although, in principle, effect modifications within subgroups should be detectable, such detection may be impossible even with very large numbers. To pool data where there is strong statistical evidence of heterogeneity will obscure real modifiers of the treatment effect (Villar et al. 1995). Second, in a large, simple, multi-centre trial there is little restriction on non-trial treatments. Where such treatments replicate the effect of intervention under test, a bias will arise that causes any true treatment effect to be underestimated. Power calculations are then meaningless, since the issue is bias rather than precision. Trial size is irrelevant to the problem of bias except to give unjustified authority to the result: the true treatment effect remains unknown!

Single-centre studies have the obvious advantage of eliminating such bias, but few would be able to recruit enough patients within a reasonable length of time. Prolonged trials of themselves, however, can present a bias in as far as investigator fatigue can develop while – with the passage of time – advances in medical management may alter or influence patient care.

The primary ICU admitting reason can be sepsis, or sepsis can be a complication in a patient receiving intensive care because of a host of underlying disorders. As study centres can range from large tertiary care teaching hospitals to smaller non-teaching community hospitals, these concurrent diseases (co-morbidities) have the potential to be treated with vastly different approaches. These differences in presentation, co-morbidities and level of care can be controlled by randomisation, but unfortunately patients are randomised within study centres and not randomly assigned between study centres. This may result in significantly different patient populations and co-morbidities at each centre receiving different treatment regimens. Thus, with a combination of a lack of randomisation between study centres, which can result in different patient populations at each centre, and the presence of different treatment regimens for co-morbidities at each centre, we have the potential for a significant bias to enter into analysis. This potential for bias is not new to most statisticians, especially to those who have performed a meta-analysis (Villar et al. 1995), but this particular form of bias has been dealt with very poorly by previous multi-centre randomised clinical trials for sepsis treatment. For the HA-1A study, for example, Warren et al. (Warren et al. 1992) have pointed out a "centre effect" with a benefit in patients with shock demonstrated only from centres with a high mortality rate. Other factors possibly biasing the outcome included the effect of inadequate or unknown antibiotic treatment, the non-linear relationship between the APACHE II score and the risk of hospital death, and the problems in predicting mortality in post-operative surgical patients and those with multiple organ failure.

5.4.
Appropriate Endpoints for Assessing Successful Adjunctive Treatment in Critically Ill Patients

There still exist many controversies not only about treatment strategies (anti-infective; anti-mediator; anti-inflammatory; suppression, augmentation or substitution of certain functions or components of the immune response) but also about the evaluation of treatment efficacy in patients with sepsis. The two problems are interdependent and cannot be discussed separately. The criteria of response to treatment may vary from one group of investigators to the next making it difficult to put the results of different studies into their proper perspective. Thus, a crucial issue in assessing the effectiveness of new promising therapeutic options is that of choosing the appropriate endpoints for evaluation.

Appropriate endpoints, however, are to be defined on the basis of the therapeutic goals of immuno-modulatory therapy. But what are the goals of adjunctive anti-infective or immuno-modulatory intervention? Is it the reversal of circulatory shock, the avoidance of the occurrence of secondary shock, a reduction in the number of organ failures or the reversal of organ failure(s)? Is it the reduction of APACHE scores, the reduction of the duration of stay in ICU or hospital? Is it the prevention of life-threatening adverse events or other intercurrent complications? Or is it mortality reduction, and if so, is it 28, 14, or 3-day mortality that is relevant? Thus, when designing a study the most appropriate endpoints have to be considered. But are the most appropriate endpoints also the clinically most relevant ones? And when contemplating the notion of clinically relevant endpoints, the question logically arises: relevant to whom? To the patient or to the therapist? And what is relevant to the patient?

Because the most common outcome in animal studies looking at treatment efficacy is mortality, and to fulfil the requirements of the "Food and Drug Administration", all major sepsis trials to date have used all-cause mortality as the primary study outcome (Sibbald and Vincent 1995 in Clinical trials…). A further reason for choosing mortality as the endpoint is that future novel adjunctive agents would be difficult to evaluate if a favourable effect on morbidity alone was to be a criterion of efficacy.

5.4.1
Pros and Cons of Mortality as Primary Endpoint in Critically Ill Patients

Although the literature on animal studies commonly cites a number of outcomes that are relevant to the study of human sepsis, mortality is the most important one (Barriere and Lowry 1995). Thus, clinical trials have usually chosen an intend-to-treat analysis of the reduction in 28- or 30-day all-cause– mortality as the primary endpoint for efficacy Also 14- or 3-day mortality has been used and might be a better test of performance than death after 28 days, because it might more accurately reflect the immuno-pharmacology of the intervention. Since mortality in sepsis is not a rare event, it does not limit effective study design. Total mortality as the primary endpoint has the undeniable, highly desirable characteristics of being unambiguous, easily measured and important (Friedmann and Schron 1992). However, patients may die as a direct result of the septic process, but also as a result of the interaction between sepsis and other pre-existing conditions, or even because of a pathologic event, not at all related to sepsis. Thus, the notion of attributable versus all-cause mortality has to be defined.

All-cause mortality ranges between 20 and 60% and represents the over-all death rate of a cohort of patients who developed bacteremic sepsis in course of their ICU or hospital stay (Gasche et al. 1995). In other words, these patients might die because of sepsis, or with sepsis but because of unrelated medical conditions, or after sepsis resolution. Attributable mortality defines the mortality rate attributed to the infection, apart from the underlying disease or other confounding factors that also might contribute to death; these patients die directly because of sepsis. Attributable mortality from nosocomial blood stream infection averages 26% in hospital wide series but varies according to the microorganisms causing the infection and the patient populations. Fatality rate is higher in critically ill ICU than in ward patients (Gasche et al. 1995).

Many agents proved to be valid modalities for treatment in animal experiments, but practically no recent study in the clinical setting has been successful using the same therapeutic approaches (Piper at al. 1996). Therefore, animal experiments have to be questioned as valid predictors of the clinical therapeutic efficacy of new treatment modalities in critically ill patients (Piper et al. 1996). Indeed, for ethical rather than scientific reasons, studies with mortality as an outcome are commonly conducted in small animals such as mice or rats. However, the results of these studies can be criticised, since it is difficult to extrapolate findings in small, endotoxin-resistant animals to patients (Redl et al. 1996). Yet there may be other reasons for failure of clinical studies to reflect the successful results from animal experiments. Examples are the need for long-term animal studies with ICU-like conditions to simulate the often delayed onset of organ dysfunction, using sepsis or organ dysfunction criteria to start the treatment instead of a fixed time schedule. New combined models should be considered where, for instance, hemorrhagic shock precedes a sepsis procedure, to avoid using healthy animals which often do not represent the ICU patient.

Although many reasons have been offered to explain the failure of phase III clinical trials which evaluate innovative approaches in the treatment of sepsis (i.e. anti-endotoxin strategies, interleukin-1 receptor antagonists, anti-tumor necrosis factor strategies), potentially important factors are the quality, quantity and interpretation of the preclinical data obtained from animal studies from which such strategies ultimately evolved (Neugebauer et al. 1998; Piper et al. 1996; Redl et al. 1996). Perhaps a more rigorous and comprehensive examination of the agents in a more relevant animal model would have prevented the premature use of a potentially harmful drug in phase III clinical trials. As shown with the HA-1A antibody studies, certain aspects cannot or can only inadequately be studied in small animals (Piper et al. 1996; Redl et al. 1996). Species-dependent differences in the cardiovascular response to sepsis need to be considered when extrapolating data from small animal studies to larger species such as humans. In the animal model, it is not possible to recreate the often complex interaction between intercurrent illness, sepsis and supportive therapy that contributes to mortality in the critically ill patient (Neugebauer et al. 1998; Piper et al. 1996; Redl et al. 1996). One commonly used supportive therapy that can be easily incorporated into animal studies is the administration of antibiotics. As a result animal studies looking at the efficacy of a given adjunctive intervention should seek to determine if efficacy is still present in antibiotic-treated animals.

In critically ill patients, the underlying disease and the functional health status are the most important determinants of outcome. In a recent report on gram-negative bacteremia, the underlying disease was found to represent the most important prognostic factor (Vincent 1995). Thus, one may expect any novel therapeutic intervention to have only a modest effect on outcome from severe sepsis (Vincent 1995).

Because of the considerable cons of mortality as an endpoint (time of assessment, death not disease-specific, insensitive to particular treatment effects, reduces complex illness to one event etc.) it has been suggested not to use all-cause mortality (28-day window) or attributable mortality as the sole endpoints, but to regard the reduction or reversal of organ failure as a valid efficacy endpoint and also to consider quality of life an important parameter (Sibbald and Vincent 1995 in Clinical trials...). New forms of therapy may not result in improvement in survival, but may reduce morbidity. A more complete and rapid reversal of organ failure or a lower complication rate may represent a major health achievement and may also reduce the treatment costs. Therefore, quality-of-life measures, surrogate measures of severity of illness, or overall costs of therapy have recently been proposed to evaluate the therapeutic efficacy of new approaches.

5.4.2
Surrogate Endpoints as an Alternative to Mortality

In recent years, there has been interest in the use of organ failure scores as a surrogate outcome in phase II and phase III clinical trials (Piper et al. 1996; Marshall 1995). Although mortality as an endpoint is characterised by some advantages, it must not be forgotten that the goal of treatment in sepsis is to preserve or improve organ function. Thus, the assessment of reduction in morbidity rather than in mortality is more and more favoured. Five organ failure descriptors have been shown to correlate with ICU mortality in a dose-dependent fashion (Marshall 1995) as does hypotension (Table 1). Such a scoring system may represent an appropriate endpoint in studies looking at therapeutic efficacy. In addition, the severity of illness score, acute organ failure and the characteristics of underlying diseases should be accounted for in outcome analysis.

Organ failure can be defined by three types of criteria: 1. Objective criteria based on measurable parameters, such as those shown in Table 1. These are by far the preferred criteria. 2. Categorical diagnoses, such as cholecystitis or ARDS. These should be avoided, as these definitions are somewhat arbitrary and subjective. 3. Criteria based on treatment, such as the level of PEEP, to define the degree of respiratory failure, the requirements for hemodialysis or hemofiltraton to define renal failure. These criteria should also be avoided, as they may critically depend on the policy of the ICU.

Organ dysfunction is frequent in sepsis and associated with a poor prognosis and outcome. New immunotherapies may prevent the development of organ dysfunction and thereby improve outcome. Reliable definitions of risk factors associated with poor outcome in sepsis are needed to help to select candidates for these expensive agents.

Table 1. Organ-specific, non-dichotomous objective descriptors of functional impairment or failure. Increasing values of at least the first five parameters have been shown to correlate with ICU mortality

Organ System	Measurable Parameter
Respiratory	PaO_2/FIO_2 ratio
Renal	Serum creatinine
Hematologic	Platelet count
Central nervous	Glasgow coma score
Hepatic	Serum bilirubin
Cardiovascular	Blood pressure
Gastrointestinal	No appropriate one

Multiple Organ Dysfunction Syndrome (MODS) as an Endpoint

The development of organ dysfunction represents more than simply the protracted process of dying despite maximal supportive care. Organ system dysfunction in critically ill patients is potentially reversible and arises from a definable group of noxious events such as infection, ischemia, or tissue injury. The introduction of the term Multiple Organ Dysfunction Syndrome (MODS) reflects that organ dysfunction comprises a clinical syndrome that has a common pathophysiological basis and is potentially amenable to specific therapeutic interventions through strategies designed to modulate the host's immune response (Marshall 1995).

Global severity of organ dysfunction during an ICU stay shows a strong correlation with ICU mortality (Marshall 1995), as well as with susceptibility to ICU-acquired infection and the expression of a clinical septic response (Rangel-Frausto et al. 1995). Similarly, graded degrees of dysfunction within given organ systems could be shown to correlate with incremental increases in ICU mortality (Marshall 1995). Such correlations have been described for PO_2/FIO_2 ratio (Murray et al. 1988), serum creatinine level (Wilson et al. 1979), serum bilirubin level (Knaus et al. 1993), platelet count (Marshall 1995), and Glasgow Coma Score (Marshall 1995). Thus, organ dysfunction in the critically ill cannot be viewed as a state or as a process, but also as an outcome, that is incorporated into the assessment of the severity of the process and is considered the worst manifestation of individual organ dysfunction during the ICU treatment.

Systems that determine the severity of MODS during an entire ICU stay may be useful as outcome measures for purposes of both research and quality assurance. As MODS is not a dichotomous event but a continuous process, two implications for the selection of descriptors of the syndrome exist: 1. Continuous variables that are preferable to dichotomous variables, and 2. the magnitude of the global organ system dysfunction which can be appropriately expressed by a score or a scale (Marshall 1995).

As already mentioned seven organ systems define MODS (Marshall 1995): The respiratory, renal, hepatic, hematologic, cardiovascular, gastrointestinal and central nervous systems (Table 1). Organ system dysfunction within these systems is best characterised by the use of single variables reflecting pathophysiologic dysfunction, (e.g. PO_2/FIO_2 ratio) rather than by variables reflecting the nature of the therapeutic intervention (need for mechanical ventilation, level of PEEP) or by composite variables (presence of ARDS, defined by hypoxemia and bilateral chest X-ray infiltrates in the absence of elevation of pulmonary capillary wedge pressure). For at least five of these systems physiologic descriptors of satisfying validity are available, only descriptors of dysfunction for the cardiovascular and the gastrointestinal system are unsatisfactory (Marshall 1995). An organ dysfunction score based on validated physiological variables can serve as a surrogate endpoint in phase II and phase III clinical trials and may also elucidate the physiologic mechanisms of action of novel therapeutic interventions. Recently, using decreased mortality along with a significant benefit in organ function has been proposed as a statistical endpoint for sepsis trials. Survival analysis (Knaus et al. 1993) uses a time to event (mortality) approach as the primary statistical endpoint for sepsis trials. A time-to-event analysis is important to consider when a therapy does not alter mortality rates, but may actually delay the onset of mortality and improve the quality-of-life experience. The primary advantage of the use of survival analysis is a small increase in statistical power compared to the direct comparison of mortality rates.

Provided that the benefit to a specific organ system has been explicitly demonstrated in previous studies, and that unambiguous easily measured and important functional definitions of organ failure are available, this approach could indeed result in fewer patients being required for definitive licensing studies. It should be noted, however, that deviations from predicted mortality using scoring systems such as APACHE, SAPS or combined organ failure scores are not sufficiently accurate or precise to warrant their use as a surrogate mortality outcome in a well designed randomised clinical trial. Also the comparison of survival of so-called responders versus non-responders is not an acceptable method for showing therapeutic efficacy. Before survival time is adopted as an endpoint, the question has to be answered whether or not a delay in mortality is clinically important and provides benefit to the patient.

5.5
Future Perspectives

As stated earlier, the clinical trial is fundamental to the assessment of new therapeutic interventions in humans. While the clinical trial must remain the standard for assessing safety and efficacy of new interventions, there are opportunities to improve the design, the execution, and the analysis of the trials (Sibbald and Vincent 1995 in clinical trials...; Murray et al. 1988). Over the past decades, no single new agent or adjunctive concept has yet demonstrated improvement of the patient's outcome in sepsis or septic shock. These disappointing result have been the subject of discussion in the literature and even pharmaceutical industry started to re-think the approach to the complex problem of sepsis in the critically ill patient (Finch 1998; Neugebauer et al. 1998; Sibbald and Vincent 1995 in Update...; Piper et al. 1996; Vincent 1995; Sibbald and Vincent 1995 in Clinical Trials...; Redl et al. 1996; Sibbald and Vincent 1995 in Round table conference...).

Treatment of sepsis remains largely supportive with emphasis on adequate antibiotic treatment and source control. Nevertheless, improved study designs are considered mandatory if future progress is to be made in the care of these patients.

The disappointing and often contradictory results of recent forays into the field of manipulation of the host inflammatory response suggest that we do not yet know which patients should receive such interventions. This underlines the need to develop models that evaluate differences in illness severity (reduced heterogeneity of study population) and strategies for the formal evaluation of the adequacy of antibiotic treatment, source control and supportive therapeutic regimens. Finally, better study designs (statistics, single versus multi-centre study; study population based on pathophysiological rather than quantitative aspects) as well as the use of more appropriate primary endpoints for the assessment of therapeutic efficacy are essential elements in this process.

5.5.1
Less Heterogeneous Study Populations

Future clinical trials will have to stratify the patients according to the severity of the disease process and thus their chances of survival. Patients with high chances of survival should be eliminated, because they are likely to do well even in the absence of additional therapy. At the other end of the spectrum, patients who are very debilitated are likely to die and should therefore not be enrolled in such study protocols. It is also important to identify the source of infection, in particular the urinary tract should be separated from the other sources of infection. Effective randomisation and blinding are obligatory to remove potential sources of bias. Randomised trials should employ a formal statistical test of baseline characteristics to determine that randomisation worked. Baseline risk assessment allows to confirm an equal risk distribution in placebo and treatment groups, and to quantify the benefits relative to the individual patients risk. Severity scores such as APACHE, SAPS, MPM should be used. The presence of proven infection has to be considered, and also types of microbial pathogens and origins of the septic process are crucial. The location of the patient as well as the duration of hospital or ICU stay at the time of the onset of sepsis (which is in most cases the time of recruitment) are also crucial. Antibiotic treatment at the time of sepsis is important, pre-existing co-morbidities must be taken into account, and the number of organ dysfunctions at onset of sepsis as well as surgical or non-surgical drainage of an abscess must be recorded.

5.5.2
Adequacy of Antibiotic Treatment, Source Control and Supportive Therapies

There is currently no formal standardised approach to the evaluation of the adequacy of antibiotic treatment and source control for clinical trials in sepsis. Such evaluations are generally performed by clinical evaluation committees on a case by case basis (Sprung et al. 1996). It is obviously important that the individuals performing these evaluations are experienced in the clinical management of these complex disease processes, and in the advantages and weaknesses of differing approaches. Recently, the exact working of such a clinical evaluation committee has been described in detail (INTERSEPT Study (Cohen and Carlet 1996). The author reported on a scientific extramural review committee (SERC) (Sprung et al. 1996; Cohen and Carlet 1996) which independently monitored a prospective international 3-arm, double-blind, placebo-controlled, randomised study of the efficacy and safety of a murin monoclonal antibody to human TNF to patients with sepsis. Of importance were the SERC assessment of the medical and surgical management, appropriateness of antibiotic treatment and the reasons for withdrawal or withholding of life-sustaining therapy, and its role in defining and analysing other unforeseen confounding events that were defined as underlying or unforeseen conditions which might seriously interfere with the potential of the therapeutic agent to produce its effects (Sprung et al. 1996).

These SERC assessments insured not only strict adherence to the protocol but also provided an independent professional assessment of the patient population, such as the nature of the underlying disease, the primary site of infection, the quality of the microbiological monitoring, the appropriateness of the antibiotic management, the overall standard of care and the "do not resuscitate" issues (Sprung et al. 1996; Cohen and Carlet 1996). As a result a more defined population of subjects was described and the therapeutic potential of the study drug could be more fairly assessed by eliminating biases which are inherent in any simple randomisation of patients such as those suffering from the sepsis syndrome.

In addition, the adequacy of source control can be evaluated by a number of complementary methods including an expert consensus, objective radiographic or microbiologic findings, and autopsy evidence. The gold standard for the evaluation of the adequacy of source control is post mortem examination. A careful post mortem examination should be undertaken in every non-survivor enrolled in clinical trials in sepsis and consent for such examination should be vigorously sought. However, none of these proposals is by itself definitive, and there is a striking paucity of published data to permit their exact evaluation.

5.5.3
Study Design (Statistics, Study Population)

Sample sizes for treatment trials with categorical outcomes are conventionally derived by balancing three elements: a difference between alternative treatments in the event rates or the outcomes of interests (clinically important difference), the alpha error tolerance (false positive risk) and the beta error tolerance (false negative risk). In the past, a tendency towards large, simple trials (mega-trials) could be observed. However, the large, simple trial is only one of several research strategies to be deployed in therapeutic research (Yusuf et al. 1994). The performance of these large trials can now be compared with other approaches in an expanding trials literature (Villar et al. 1995). Its particular value is in the detection of small treatment effects which are likely to be uniform across patient subgroups, not highly sensitive to protocol details and not replicated by non-trial therapy (Yusuf et al. 1984).

Such a mega-trial should, first, specify treatment conditions, e.g. timing, dosing, regimen, that are likely to produce the maximum treatment effect. It is not surprising that the details of the dosing regimen can also alter the true treatment effect, and it is therefore essential to have mechanistic and pathophysiologic insights from experimental models and exploratory human studies when designing such a large trial. This was not always the case in previous trials on adjunctive immunotherapy of sepsis.

Second, the true treatment effect should be estimated with a minimum of bias and an adequate precision. Effective randomisation and objective endpoints are necessary but not sufficient in themselves to control bias. When recruitment is distributed over many hundreds of centres and may outweigh the potential power gain of increased patient numbers, the contrast between treatment and placebo is blurred by non-trial therapy, or there is a non-differential inaccuracy of data, including misclassification.

Where there is insufficient existing knowledge to support the underlying assumptions, adequately powered conventional trials with more restrictive protocols and fuller patient data are preferable. Validity must take precedence over power in the design process.

As a general principle, the primary analysis of any randomised controlled trial must be performed on an intention-to-treat basis (Doig and Rochon 1995). This means, that as soon as the patient is randomised to a treatment arm, the patient is considered to have entered the study and must be included in the primary analysis whether or not the treatment is successfully completed. As the trial size is irrelevant to the problem of bias, it only gives unjustified authority to the result, thus, it could be wise to choose a well defined patient group for a single-centre study with a very restrictive protocol instead of believing in the power of big numbers. In principle, to maximise the chances of success of a novel therapeutic intervention, clinical trials may follow two different approaches: the first one is to include a very large number of patients into clinical trials that confounding factors will be eventually eliminated (Doig and Rochon 1995). But a too large clinical trial may mask the evidence of a beneficial effect in a subgroup of patients if this therapy has deleterious effects in another subgroup. The second approach is to focus any new therapeutic intervention on a very specific group of patients with a clearly identifiable disease process. Rather than mixing patients with different stages of organ failure or different co-morbidities or different underlying pathophysiologies, these trials would include well-defined groups of patients.

5.5.4
Appropriate Primary Endpoints

In general, outcomes should be clinically relevant, reproducible, specified a-priori, and should include both measures of benefit and harm. Besides the primary endpoints, all patient outcomes, withdrawals, drop-outs, success and failure rates should be reported. As long as no other endpoints are available, clinical trials of sepsis should make use of clinical endpoints. Clinical endpoints have the advantage of defining clinical utility. As outlined in the respective chapter above, all-cause mortality is not considered the most appropriate clinical endpoint and should be replaced by surrogate parameters with or without survival analysis.

There is also a very useful way of summarising the efficacy of an intervention and of evaluating the impact of therapy: the Number Needed to Treat. This concept describes the number of patients that one would need to treat to prevent one event (Cook 1995 in Clinical trials...). A relative risk reduction may be quite impressive, but if the baseline risk of this clinical endpoint is low, the impact of treatment may be minimal. Although a therapy may be very efficacious, it may not be an efficient utilisation of resources both in terms of the resources needed to implement the therapy and also of the potential side effects. If the clinical endpoint studied occurs in a low rate, than the number needed to treat may be large. In this context, the costs of an expensive therapy would result in the expenditure of scarce resources.

Therefore, costs are not an appropriate study endpoint. An economic evaluation is most appropriately conducted and most useful, when it is preceded by 3 other types of evaluation which address different but essential complementary questions: Can it work? Does it work? Is it reaching those who need it (Cook 1995 in Economic evaluation...) Economic evaluations attempt to identify and to make explicit one set of criteria which may be useful in deciding among different uses of scarce resources. An economic evaluation is a comparative analysis of alternative courses of action in terms of both their costs and consequences. The task of an economic analysis is therefore to identify, measure, value and compare the costs and consequences of the alternatives being considered. Cost-benefit analysis should be conducted when quality-of-life was the primary or one of the primary endpoints, or when it is desirable to combine both morbidity and mortality (Cook 1995 in Economic evaluation...).

References

American College of Chest Physicians/Society of Critical Care Medicine Consensus Conference Committee (1992) ACCP/SCCM Consensus Conference: Definitions for sepsis and organ failure and guidelines for the use of innovative therapies in sepsis. Crit Care Med 20: 864–874

Barriere SL, Lowry SF (1995) An overview of mortality risk prediction in sepsis. Crit Care Med 23: 376-393

Baumgartner JD, Bula C, Vaney C, Wu MM, Eggimann P, Perret C (1992) A novel score for predicting the mortality of septic shock patients. Crit Care Med 20: 953–960

Beam TR Jr, Gilbert DN, Kunin CM (1992) General guidelines for the clinical evaluation of anti-infective drug products. Clin Infect Dis 15 (Suppl 1): S 5–32

Beam TR Jr, Gilbert DN, Kunin CM (1993) European guidelines for anti-infective drug products. Clin Infect Dis 17: 787–788

Bone RC (1991) A critical evaluation of new agents for the treatment of sepsis. JAMA 266: 1686–1691

Bone RC (1993) Gram-negative sepsis: a dilemma of modern medicine. Clin Microbiol Rev 6: S7–68

Bone RC, Fisher CJ, Clemmer TP, Slotman GJ, Metz CA, Balk RA (1989) Sepsis syndrome: a valid clinical entity. Crit Care Med 17: 389–393

Bone RC, Sprung CL, Sibbald WJ (1992) Definitions for sepsis and organ failure. Crit Care Med 20: 724–725

Brun-Buisson C, Doyon F, Carlet J et al. (1995) Incidence, risk factors and outcome of severe sepsis and septic shock in adults. JAMA 274: 968–974

Cohen J, Carlet J (1996) INTERSEPT: an international multicenter placebo-controlled trial of monoclonal antibody to human tumor necrosis factor alpha in patients with sepsis. Crit Care Med 24: 1431–1440

Cook DJ (1995) Clinical trials in the treatment of sepsis: An evidence-based approach. In: Clinical trials for the treatment of sepsis. Sibbald WJ, Vincent JL (Eds) Berlin, Springer-Verlag, pp XIX

Cook DJ (1995) Economic evaluation in the critical care literature. In: Clinical trials for the treatment of sepsis. Sibbald WJ, Vincent JL (Eds) Berlin, Springer-Verlag, pp 370

Doig GS, Rochon J (1995) Statistical considerations for the design of the optimal clinical trial. In: Clinical trials for the treatment of sepsis. Sibbald WJ, Vincent JL (Eds) Berlin, Springer-Verlag, pp 345

Finch RG (1998) Design of clinical trials in sepsis: problems and pitfalls. J Antimicrob Chemother 41 (Suppl. A): 95–102

Friedmann LM, Schron EB (1992) Statistical problems in the design of antiarrhythmic drug trials. J Cardiovasc Pharm 20 (Suppl. 2): S 114–S118

Gasche Y, Pittet D, Suter PM (1995) Outcome and prognostic factors in bacteremic sepsis. In: Clinical trials for the treatment of sepsis. Sibbald WJ, Vincent JL (Eds) Berlin, Springer-Verlag, pp 35

Guyatt GH, Sackett DL, Cook DJ (1994) Users' guides to the medical literature. II. How to use an article about therapy or prevention. JAMA 271: 59–63

Immunocompromised Host Society (1990) The design, analysis and reporting of clinical trials on the empirical antibiotic management of the neutropenic patient. Report of a consensus panel. J Infect Dis 161: 397–401

Knaus WA, Draper EA, Wagner DP, Zimmerman JE (1985) APACHE II: A severity of disease classification system. Crit Care Med 13: 818–829

Knaus WA, Harrell FE, Fisher CJ et al. (1993) The clinical evaluation of new drugs for sepsis. A prospective study design based on survival analysis. JAMA 270: 1233–1241

Knaus WA, Wagner DP, Harrell FE (1995) What determines prognosis in sepsis? In: Clinical trials for the treatment of sepsis. Sibbald WJ, Vincent JL (Eds) Berlin, Springer-Verlag, pp 141

Kreger BE, Craven DE, McCabe WR (1980) Gram-negative bacteremia. IV: Re-evaluation of clinical features and treatment in 612 patients. Am J Med 68: 344–355

Marshall JC (1995) Multiple organ dysfunction syndrome (MODS). In: Clinical trials for the treatment of sepsis. Sibbald WJ, Vincent JL (Eds.) Berlin, Springer-Verlag, pp 122

Murray JF, Matthay MA, Luce JM, Flick MR (1988) An expanded definition of the adult respiratory distress syndrome. Am Rev Respir Dis 138: 720–723

Neugebauer E, Rixen D, Raum M, Schäfer U (1998) Thirty years of anti-mediator treatment in sepsis and septic shock – what have we learned? Langenbeck's Arch Surg 383: 26–34

Oxman AD, Sackett DL, Guyatt GH (1993) Users' guides to the medical literature. I. How to get started. JAMA 270: 2093–2095

Piper RD, Cook DJ, Bone RC, Sibbald WJ (1996) Introducing critical appraisal to studies of animal models investigating novel therapies in sepsis. Crit Care Med 24: 2059–2070

Pittet D, Thiévent B, Wenzel RP, Li N, Gurman G, Suter PM (1993) Importance of pre-existing co-morbidities for prognosis of septicemia in critically ill patients. Int Care Med 19: 265–272

Rangel-Frausto MS, Pittet D, Costigan M et al. (1995) The natural history of the systemic inflammatory response syndrome (SIRS). JAMA 273: 117–123

Redl H, Schlag G, Bahrami S, Yao YM (1996) Animal models as the basis of pharmacologic intervention in trauma and sepsis patients. World J Surg 20: 487–492

Schwartz DB, Bone RC, Balk RA, Szidon JP (1989) Hepatic dysfunction in the adult respiratory distress syndrome. Chest 95: 871–875

Sibbald WJ, Vincent JL (1995) Round table conference on clinical trials for the treatment of sepsis. Crit Care Med 23: 394–399

Sibbald WJ, Vincent JL (1995) Round table conference on clinical trials for the treatment of sepsis. Brussels, 12-14 March 1994. Int Care Med 21: 184–189

Sibbald WJ, Vincent JL (Eds) (1995) Clinical trials for the treatment of sepsis. Update in intensive care and emergency medicine, Vol. 19, Berlin, Springer-Verlag

Sprung CL, Finch RG, Thijs LG, Glauser MP (1996) International sepsis trial (INTERSEPT): Role and impact of a clinical evaluation committee. Crit Care Med 24: 1441–1447

Villar J, Carroli G, Belizàn JM (1995) Predictive ability of meta-analyses of randomised controlled trials. Lancet 345: 772–776

Vincent JL (1995) The "at risk" patient population. In: Clinical trials for the treatment of sepsis. Sibbald WJ, Vincent JL (Eds) Berlin, Springer-Verlag, pp 13

Warren HS, Dann RL, Munford RS (1992) Anti-endotoxin monoclonal antibodies. N Engl J Med 326: 1153-1157

Wilson RF, Soullier G, Antonenko D (1979) Creatinine clearance in critically ill surgical patients. Arch Surg 114: 461-467

Yusuf S, Collins R, Peto R (1984) Why do we need some large, simple randomized trials? Stat Med 3: 409-420

Subject Index